About the Author

Allison Schleef was born, raised and lives in Mount Gambier (home of the world famous Blue Lake) in South Australia, Australia. After twenty-three years of working in the hospitality industry as a chef, Allison is enjoying her new role of stay at home mum; which also now gives her time to indulge in her small hobby business 'Little Treasures By Allison'. Sharing a mutual passion for Jack Russell Terriers with her husband, they are active within the JRTCA and Allison is a state representative for, and a long serving member of, the JRTCA's national committee.

This book is dedicated to my Son…

…My Inspiration and reason for Being; and my greatest achievement to date.
Finally, I know the meaning of Life.
XXXX

And to my dad…
My Hero, My Guiding Light XXX

And also my husband…
…For Better, For Worse XX

ALSO,
I would like to share the love with every mumma
Who has gone through a premature birth / neonatal journey,
As well as those mummas weathering their own personal storm.

Allison Schleef

A GIRAFFE CALLED NEO

AUSTIN MACAULEY
PUBLISHERS LTD.

A CIP catalogue record for this title is available from the British Library.

ISBN 978 1 78455 838 3 (Paperback)
ISBN 978 1 78455 839 0 (Hardback)

www.austinmacauley.com

First Published (2015)
Austin Macauley Publishers Ltd.
25 Canada Square Canary Wharf
London
E14 5LB

Printed and bound in Great Britain

Acknowledgements/Honourable Mentions:

A shout out must go to these people who directly or indirectly had something to do with either helping me through one of the most trying times in my entire life, or had something to do with my vision and inspiration of A GIRAFFE CALLED NEO…

My husband Paul – for standing by me, even after seeing me at my worst.

To the endless rotation of NICU Nurses and Paediatric Consultants and Neonatologists at Flinders – without you all, my Son would not be.

All my Neonatal 'Sisters from another Mister' – but especially Natalie, Kirsty, Tashii, Sharni, and Karri Anne; for their ongoing friendship.

Ange – my devoted sister, for all her kindred support.

Jen – my 'Sanity Saviour' while we were in Flinders, now my admired advocate for Premature Birth Support.

My mum and dad – for their devoted and unwavering benevolence when I needed it the most.

Marie – who never once doubted my prose and capabilities.

Sarah - my unassuming late night shoulder to cry on.

Rob – THE "Legend" of Daddy's Little Legend, and a true inspiration to me.

And to the Austin Macauley Board of Editors and my Publishing Consultant – for this incredible opportunity.

Thank you, One and All. XXXX

"The darkest hour is just before the Dawn"

– Thomas Fuller.

(Meaning: There IS Hope, even in the worst circumstances ….)

INTRODUCTION

"IF I SAID TO YOU RIGHT NOW, THAT YOU HAVE POST-NATAL DEPRESSION – HOW DOES THAT MAKE YOU FEEL?"

This was a question posed to me by my Doctor.

I sat there for a while, thinking about it. I'd heard the whispers about women with PND. I knew of the stigma attached to it. So being told point blank by my trusted health professional that it was in HER medical opinion that I was indeed suffering from it – how DID I feel, exactly?

Did I feel like the cliché – dirty and tainted? No.

Did I feel embarrassed or ashamed? No.

There was only one thing I was feeling at that particular moment – and it was overwhelming and suffocating. I felt BROKEN. Beaten down. But also, oddly, at the same time I felt relieved. Relieved that the helplessness and despair I was feeling actually had a name; that there was a valid reason. That I WASN'T going insane.

Let me introduce myself.

My name is Allison, and I have medically diagnosed Postnatal Depression.

There. It's out.

It does not mean I am a nutter. I am an ordinary woman; a daughter, a sister, a wife, a mother. I don't feel embarrassed to admit my condition. Nor do I feel ashamed by it. In fact – I feel COMPELLED to talk about it, discuss it; because from what I have experienced – and are still going through; I hope to give others comfort and strength, and, through my writing I also hope to better understand it myself, what it IS I am going through; and to hopefully educate mainstream society and create more public awareness and greater acceptance; and put an end to the ignorance.

This book is in no way a medical journal. And I point out right here and now – I am no expert on the subject. I have never professed nor pretended that I am, and I didn't write this book to be viewed upon as a Guide; however – I DID write it for the edification of others, for the empowerment and personal improvement it may give. I am honestly, openly and humbly sharing my OWN thoughts, feelings, perceptions and opinions based on my OWN experience and personal battle with PND; with the goal of my voice being heard on behalf of all women everywhere.

Statistics are that 1 in 7 mums are diagnosed with medically recognisable Postnatal Depression, and it's indiscriminate where and who it strikes. There are a range of factors that can trigger PND – Biological, Psychological and Sociocultural; and sometimes, if you're lucky, there is a catalyst, a KNOWN reason; but for the majority of the time, there is no known reason. It just IS.

But contrary to popular belief, Postnatal Depression is NOT a dirty word.

There is so much negative and unfounded stigma associated with PND, and sadly – UNFAIRLY – women are made to feel like it's some sort of shameful secret and Taboo subject that should not be spoken about; much less admitted to suffering from it; lest you be shunned by society and labelled.

Most women suffering with PND are, on the outside, perfectly NORMAL. That is, for the most part, means that we function quite well in public and even play nicely with others! HOW ABOUT THAT?!

We are women who pay the bills. Do the grocery shopping. We run errands. Chauffer the kids around town. Yes! We can drive a CAR! We put the daily meals on the table, and ensure the clothes on our family's backs are clean.

We vote. We go to work. Yes – some of us even have JOBS!

We can also hold a meaningful and coherent conversation. And that lady flashing the mega-watt smile that seems to have it all? The one you always secretly aspire to BE like? Guess What? SHE has PND!! Now WHO would have thought it, huh? And yet – she's still HER; someone that you, and all those around her, admire.

So you see – having PND, whilst being a medically recognised condition, DOESN'T mean you are a crazy lady. And, depending on your own personal views of public disclosure; doesn't mean you have to keep your condition a secret. Agreed, in absolute extreme cases it can be severely debilitating; but the good news is – it CAN be effectively treated and managed, and the sooner the diagnosis, the earlier the treatment and faster the recovery.

Postnatal Depression is more prevalent than most would care to realise. And I dare say, There are a lot of women out there who are undiagnosed as such and struggling from day to day, due largely to not knowing in the first instance how to recognise it; and then not knowing where to go from there, because they want to keep it to themselves out of fear of perceived repercussions – and from fear of being socially ostracised. I think it's absolutely abhorrent the way mainstream society have shaped the way most women are made to feel about Postnatal Depression, all because it falls into the category of 'Mental Health'. It is the ignorant and the uneducated that shun such a condition; and human nature that singles out and highlights with ridicule and malice, that of which we don't fully understand. This ignorance dates back to the 1800s, and even further – as it is documented that Postnatal Depression was recognised back as early as Hippocrates. But it was seen to be an infliction of 'melancholy, mania and hysteria', thought to stem from a supposed disorder of the reproductive system'. ('Hysteria' comes from the Greek word 'hysteron', meaning womb).

Did you know, in the Victorian Era of the 1800s, women who were diagnosed with ' Puerperal Insanity ' , later called Postnatal Depression, were more often than not sent to lunatic asylums to recuperate, and dangerous drugs such as mercury and antimony (a chemical in fire retardants!) were administered, to keep the manic patient 'nauseated' and thus less likely to 'act out'? And it was widely thought that women with PND were thought to have Cerebral Congestion and needing to have their blood cooled and thinned – so the barbarous method of 'Bleeding' the stricken woman with leeches was practised? Can you IMAGINE our civil liberties being subjected to such harsh and despotic treatments?? Luckily for us, the turn of the century saw such arbitrary and disagreeable methods abolished, and in the late 1980s there was a resurgence of Postnatal Depression Awareness and its impact on the families of those suffering from it and its effect on society in general. Just because we are women does not mean we are socially inferior, and we certainly should not be treated with such vehemence and disregard.

The state of our mental health is the same as any other part of our health – man or woman – which needs to be nurtured and maintained – so none of us need to be ashamed about it. And even though we have come a long way since the 1800s – public acceptance and awareness of PND is still grossly inadequate. Even today, if you are a woman suffering with it, you are still held in disdain and scorned, to a degree.

If society as a whole was to be honest with itself, the majority would be suffering from SOME form of mental health issue in SOME form or another. None of us are perfect. Everyone has an Achilles Heel. But no one wants to address that. Or bring it to the fore. We would much rather put our game face on, and struggle in private. Oh, to be the perfect human!

10–15 % of all mums will get a Postnatal DISORDER in some form or other.

That's 1 in every 10 mums. But a more recent study suggests that figure to be closer to 1 in every 4.

There are 3 types of Post Natal DISORDERS: The 'BABY BLUES', a brief period of emotional distress, which occurs 3–10 days after delivery in up to 80% of all women that give birth. The 'blues' is caused by several factors including sudden changes in hormone levels after childbirth, anxiety and sleep deprivation. The BABY BLUES is a transient state and generally disappears within a few days.

POSTNATAL PHYCHOSIS, a rare and severe postnatal disorder; affects only 1–3 out of every 1000 mothers.

And POSTNATAL DEPRESSION, often confused with and mistaken for the Baby Blues; however, there are important differences between the two. In PND, the symptoms are more pronounced, more severe and last a lot longer. Between 10–20 % of all women who give birth will suffer from PND to SOME degree, which can develop following the birth of ANY child – not just after the birth of the first.

Every woman suffering from PND will have her own host of symptoms, which will present and vary in severity for each individual; but common symptoms can include: Feeling 'teary' for no apparent reason, feeling low, feeling anxious or unexplained sadness, having feelings of 'worthlessness and failings' of being a good Mother; resentment, anger, irritability, confusion, lack of concentration, ongoing exhaustion not linked to sleep deprivation, weight loss or gain, loss of libido. Women often feel guilt and shame that they feel this way at a time when they should be happy, joyful and fulfilled; so all these strange conflicting feelings only magnify an already intense sense of inadequacy and general inability to cope. And this might even make you start to be socially withdrawn.

Many people automatically think that to be suffering with PND means you are at greater risk of harming your child, but that's very rarely the case. Most Mother's with PND generally have the where – with-all to look after and care for and Love their child/children just as well as any other Mother. The exception here, from what I have read, would be a Mum with severe Postnatal Psychosis, who may, THEN, present as a danger to her child, due to the delusional state of said psychosis. I would like to think that THIS form of Postnatal Disorder would be quickly recognised by a health professional and treated accordingly, but my observations in this book are based on Postnatal DEPRESSION, not Psychosis. I wouldn't feel comfortable discussing and projecting on such a topic any further when it isn't part of what I myself have experienced. Misinformation could be detrimental to someone suffering from such a severe condition.

Sadly though, there are women who have felt so desolate and overwhelmed that they have taken their own life, because they have felt like they had nowhere to turn and have hit rock bottom. In fact, the noted leading cause of maternal deaths is suicide. That reality is incredibly sobering. Imagine feeling SO isolated in your own little insular existence and trapped by your own grief and sadness that you see no way forward, no way out? This is why, no matter which end of the depressive scale you happen to land on – you need to seek help.

Another interesting and little known fact is that MEN can ALSO suffer from Postnatal Depression.

Yes, you just read correctly! It is a recognised condition and is very real as well for our male counterparts. If I myself had not been diagnosed with PND and set about educating myself about it – I would never have known this.

3-10% of new dads suffer from what is known as 'Paternal PND'. It presents itself in roughly the same manner as in women, and is commonly found to begin before the birth of the baby, increasing in severity between 6 weeks and 6 months after the baby is born, with minimal recovery by the end of the first year.

As with women, the causes are many and varied, and PND in the mother is a strong predictor of partners having it too (but is not always the case), with the most noted leading triggers of PND in men being:

- the impact of changing roles in the family (more responsibility on the shoulders of the father, i.e.: extra financial burden),

- stress and changes in the dynamics of the relationship,

- having difficulty adjusting to the transition to parenthood,

- general lack of social and emotional support,

- and unmet prenatal expectations.

Whilst my writing is aimed mostly at women, Men should not take their condition lightly either. New fathers don't have the access to the sort of services afforded to new mothers after childbirth, hence the reason why men slip unnoticed under the radar.

While it is important that we, as women, have some understanding of what factors may have put us at risk of PND – determining the causes should not become the sole focus. TREATMENT should be.

And it is my belief that greater recognition of PND will hopefully encourage women to seek help early; and by creating awareness of PND within our society, it will hopefully lead to an improved understanding and acceptance of the illness in general. Having PND does not and should not make you a social pariah.

And trust me – you are no less of a mother if you have it, and certainly no less of a woman if you are suffering from it. Furthermore, acknowledging it and seeking treatment does not make you weak; In fact, it takes COURAGE to put your hand up and say "I'm struggling – I need help". And if YOU can't see it personally, hopefully your partner, friends or family CAN recognise it, and help you get the help you need.

With the right support network, and medical treatment, your life can continue on with minimal interference and your world can be a better place.

CHAPTER ONE

In order for you to relate to my experience, I would like to share with you what I believe was the 'catalyst' for MY Postnatal Depression.

Let me take you on a personal sojourn that inevitably changed my whole life; a journey which is not isolated to just myself but to thousands of other mother's – thus highlighting and explaining and putting into perspective HOW Postnatal Depression can so easily come about.

Because I also strongly believe that the TRIGGER for my Postnatal Depression goes hand in hand with each other, and it's also another subject that also needs to be bought to light and better understood.

I'm referring to PREMATURE BIRTH.

And after you have read the brevity of my experience regarding both situations, you will understand when I say the two subjects are totally relative to each other; albeit in an encumbering way, and I think it is prudent to discuss the consequences that each issue poses, long term.

It all started for me when I gave birth prematurely at just 28 weeks gestation.

I had no medical issues with my pregnancy that I knew of. No HELLP Syndrome (the medical name given to a serious complication in pregnancy involving a combination of liver and blood disorders), no PE (Pre-Eclampsia, a pregnancy disorder characterised by high blood pressure, fluid retention and large amounts of protein in the urine), no Gestational Diabetes, No Placental Previa or Percreta – I didn't even fit into the category for pPROM (preterm premature rupture of membranes)... I suffered with NONE of these usual and common reasons for a premature birth; in fact, no NOTHING of ANY sort to explain WHY my baby decided one morning to make a hasty exit well before his due date. And I think I can safely say, THIS is what put me more at risk of ending up with Postnatal Depression after my whole ordeal. I'm not saying I WOULDN'T have suffered with it had the turn of events been completely different. Mums of Term babies get Postnatal Depression, too. But I DO believe it pretty much clinched the deal for me AS a result of what I went through. So I decided to write about my personal Premmie/Neonatal experience in the hope that it may help even just ONE mum in the future... in fact, I wrote a book about it and it was self-published in December 2013, titled BORN TOO SOON.

I know that if I had of been more informed about what COULD happen with my pregnancy, birth and baby; I may have been more prepared emotionally for what was to come. But I was naïve and blissfully unaware. And it hit me like a freight train with no brake. In the city, you are lucky enough to get a tour of a Neonatal Ward in your antenatal class. But for us folk in the country, we don't have that luxury of forewarned insight.

So what made me think MY story was something of substance to share with complete strangers? How is MY experience any different to anyone else's? Am I full of my own self-importance for having done so? Hardly, no. I am fully aware that I am not the first person to have ever had a premature baby, nor will I be the last. I did not write my book for sympathy, and our experience does not set my child on a higher plane than anyone else's. Nor does it make me an expert in the matter, or any better than any other Premmie mum.

And because of the MANY and VARIED complexities surrounding a premature baby – I openly admit there is still a LOT that I don't understand, because not everyone experiences the SAME journey or issues as the next person. Every Neonatal journey is unique; the outcome determined by the fragility and health of EACH individual prem baby.

I simply wanted to reach out to other Mums going through a similar experience, to let them know they are not alone. Until I had my premmie baby, I never knew HOW many Mum's out there – and especially in MY immediate community ALONE – had travelled this same road, and it was sort of comforting to know there were others around me who had; like safety in numbers, so to speak. 'The 'Kindred Club' you automatically become a part of without knowing it. The premmie community is a very close knit sect, very welcoming and supportive of each other.

And after the overwhelming positive response I received from my BORN TOO SOON Book Launches, it was clear that my decision to share my premmie story WAS helping other Mums.

I had strangers coming up to me and giving me a hug; and being told how inspirational I was to be brave enough to speak out about something so personal has encouraged me to keep going in my quest to highlight these two subjects, and the detrimental and devastating effects they can have on your life, because there is no contingency plan when it comes to giving birth prematurely. It's not something that you counted on.

And no one knows whether YOU will be one of the women that Postnatal Depression decides to pay a visit to. It's a demographic lottery.

If there are any pregnant ladies reading this, please know my intention is NOT to scare you.

Unfortunately though, this IS the reality of what all pregnant women ARE at risk of facing. Statistically speaking, approximately 80% of Preterm Births are not anticipated.

We get pregnant, and then we giddily plan the months ahead, with a distinct vision in mind and expectations of how things are going to pan out. But for some, it doesn't happen the way we thought it would. Some of us find ourselves in the most frightening outcome that even in our wildest dreams, we couldn't have imagined.

And it happens to a lot of us without any prior warning.

Indeed, some Mums have a much more traumatic journey than others, but at the end of the day – ANY deviation from what YOU had envisioned the birth of YOUR precious baby to be, is going to have a profound effect on you – ESPECIALLY if it has involved a Neonatal Admission. And whether your baby is there for 1 day, 1 week, 1 month or several – the length of their stay is irrelevant; you still suffer the same grief, the same sense of loss, the same feelings of having no control, the overwhelming feelings of failure, and of being ripped of (of) what was meant to have been, a beautiful experience.

Put simply – if you give birth and cannot hold your new-born straight away (or even for DAYS after, like I couldn't), cannot feed your baby the conventional way (either breast or bottle), do not have the freedom to even pick up and cuddle your baby at will, and cannot take your baby home with you when you go… and then to ALSO have to Watch your precious baby be subjected to the barrage of daily tests and procedures, and to witness them having to fight on a daily basis for even the simple right to BREATHE that we all take for granted – it's crushing to the soul; absolutely emotionally debilitating.

For those Mums who HAVE been lucky enough to HAVE carried their babies to Term, and had a day or two in hospital before going home with your healthy little gurgling bundle – THIS is the other side of the coin. The side no-one tells you about, before the fact.

For those who have never experienced the emotional ravages of a Premature Birth, you don't understand how MUCH and how BIG every milestone thereafter IS for us, and the importance of what it means. I guess it's like cancer – once you have been touched by it personally, it changes you. Everything about it consumes you. You want to understand it, you want to make OTHERS understand it, and want others to know what it's like for you to be dealing WITH it. It's the same for having had a Prem Baby.

Although the journey in BORN TOO SOON was MINE, something I lived and endured; even those family members that were there WITH me at the time, didn't WALK it with me completely. How could they? How can ANYONE possibly understand what it is truly like, unless they have BEEN THERE themselves? I firmly believe a little knowledge goes a long way, and in hindsight I really wish I had known IN ADVANCE what was potentially in store for me BEFORE I was thrust into my seemingly never-ending nightmare. Not that it would have made the journey any easier or the pain any less.

But at least if I HAD known about it, I wouldn't have been so totally blindsided by it when it happened. I honestly believe it should be part of EVERY Antenatal curriculum – whether you reside in the city OR the country. I mean, they cover the pain and indignation of trying to push a watermelon out of a hole the size only a small plum (in all reality!) could come out of, and go into great detail the horrors of epidurals and C-sections and episiotomies... Why not at the very least, TOUCH on the subject of Premature Birth, instead of just coyly alluding to it? It's a very REAL possibility of every pregnancy – even more so for those deemed with high risk pregnancies – and something every expectant Mum-to-be needs to know about and be aware of.

So I decided to share my maternal heartaches and struggles, as intimate as they may be, with the intention of educating future mummies about to embark on their own Neonatal journey, and to offer comfort and hope should they need it (which they will). There is a whole community of graduate Neonate babies and parents out there – take heart, YOU ARE NEVER ALONE.

I would also like to think my writing may be an inspiration to other Neo mums doing it tough; to reassure them that it's not ALL heartache and tears. These babies are truly one of life's little miracles; and looking back, I am in awe of their resilience and fighting spirit. I think the babies are sometimes stronger than their mummies. They may bear the physical scars of the telltale procedures they underwent, but WE bear the mental scars on their behalf.

In the next Chapter, before I launch into my soliloquy, I will start with some facts about Premature Birth and babies that I gleaned from reputable Government websites. If you or anyone in your family have never been touched by the experience of a premature birth, this information will hopefully give you an appreciation of what a harrowing and life altering situation it really is. Because the humbling statistics are, each year, 15 million babies are born too soon worldwide. In Australia ALONE, 25,000 babies are born too soon EACH YEAR. That's roughly 8% of all babies born annually, or 1 in every 12 babies. Roughly 11.4% of all pregnancies end in premature birth. And a further 1 in 6 babies require the specialist care of a Neonatal Unit at birth, prem or not.

The ubiquitous nature of premature birth is greater than most people would care to think; but it's not widely talked about – and after personally going through it, I think it's because of the sombre and delicate shroud that surrounds a prem baby, and the ignorance and ambivalence some people have toward it due to being uneducated about it.

And I don't mean that in a derogatory way, either. FOR EXAMPLE: I can vividly remember a comment made to me by someone just after we had come Home from our long hospital stay. This person came up to us in the supermarket, looked into the capsule at my son Aidan and flippantly said, "He's still alive, then". That remark cut me to the core. I was dumbfounded and numb that someone could be so insensitive to what had been the most traumatic and frightening experience of my life.

Another time, someone said to me after seeing Aidan for the first time: "Oh! But he *looks* just like a normal BABY!!!???????" I felt like asking – "Well, what were you expecting – a two-headed ALIEN??!!"

I was also asked (in a conversation and totally out of innocent curiosity – of which I didn't take offence to) … What did I think when I looked at my new-born prem baby? Was I shocked and disgusted by his appearance? Or did I think he was as beautiful as any other new-born?

It is true, premature babies DO look physically different. There is no denying that fact.

For crying out loud – they are still developing!!! But when I saw my son for the first time, I was overcome with so much love for him, and instinctively went into a fierce maternal protective mode; so much so that I think if anyone HAD made such a reference to his looks at the time, I would have launched myself at them with teeth bared and claws out, ready for a bloodied battle. To me, he was perfection.

I know these comments weren't said in malice – they were said in complete ignorance because these people simply didn't know any better, and they don't know what to say when confronted with it . But it just proves my point that people with no knowledge about prem babies really have no idea. In this case, ignorance really IS bliss.

I openly admit – until I went through it, I didn't have a clue about Prems and Neonatal Units and how it affects those involved, either. So until it *happened* to ME – I was just as blissfully ignorant.

And if you have never experienced it first-hand, you will never TRULY understand what it's like; or the enormity of the emotional roller-coaster you are forced to ride without your prior consent. But for those who have, it's something you will NEVER forget. In time, the pain of remembering it may lessen somewhat, and you may even be able to reflect back on it without the torrent of tears, but it will always be lodged in your mind. You will look back months – even YEARS, later – at photos of your new-born, and instead of appraising the studio photographic art you had planned to commission of your baby, dressed in the latest infant couture and cute poses; you have vivid memories in their place of your baby starkly dressed in just a nappy with all the tubing and lifesaving paraphernalia over the face and body. This is how most Neo Mums will remember their premmies… but it's in no way any less beautiful. In fact, one of my most favourite photos of my son is a close up of him in his isolette, complete with facial hardware to boot. It's how I viewed him daily for months, and it was my lot in life, as such; so you kind of subconsciously accept the situation for what it is, even though to see your tiny baby inside a plastic bubble – an artificial womb – hooked up to life saving machines; is one of the most humbling, numbing, confronting thing you are most likely to ever experience. The feeling of total failure and utter helplessness is overwhelming and all consuming.

Knowing there is nothing you can do to make things better; only wait it out, hour by hour, day by day, and hope and pray that the final outcome for your frail baby will be a good one. Because sadly, not all premmie outcomes are good. Despite the advances in medical marvels and perinatal care, approximately 1 million of the babies born premature (worldwide) lose their life battle. So for ME, on reflection (and as they say – hindsight is a wonderful thing), any and ALL memories I have of my son in the NICU are good ones, despite the intense emotions that may accompany them.

I should also add here, that it's not JUST the mum's who have had premature babies that are profoundly affected by a Neonatal experience.

It's also the mums who HAVE been lucky enough to have had a full-term pregnancy; But their baby has been born with a medical condition, complication or illness which has seen them admitted to a Neonatal Ward … Basically, any deviation from what we expect to be a "normal" birth experience with a "normal" homecoming.

CHAPTER TWO

Pre-term birth is the leading cause of new-born deaths (within the first 4 weeks of life),

And the 2nd leading cause of death, after pneumonia, in children under 5 years of age.

The WORLD HEALTH ORGANISATION (W.H.O) defines Prematurity as "Babies born before 37 weeks from the first day of the last menstrual period".

At the time of writing, the latest Australian Mothers and Babies Report was that 79% of Babies were born between 32 & 36 weeks; 10% were born between 28 & 31 weeks, and 11% were born at or LESS than 28 weeks.

45–50 % of Preterm Births are idiopathic (that is, no known cause). 30 % are related to PPROM. And 15 – 20% are attributed to medically indicated causes. That's quite a sobering thought – that nearly half of all prem births happen for no known reason.

For those that don't already know, there are 3 Categories of Prematurity:

-   MODERATELY PRETERM, for babies born between 32 to under 37 weeks gestation,

-   EXTREME PRETERM, for babies born between 26 to under 32 weeks gestation, and

- MICRO PRETERM, for babies born at 25 weeks gestation and below.

There are also 3 Categories of BIRTH WEIGHT for Prems:
- A baby born weighing less than 2500gm is considered to be in the LOW weight range.

- A baby born weighing less than 1500gm is considered to be in the VERY LOW range.

- And a baby born weighing less than 1000gm is in the EXTREMELY LOW weight range.

Thirty years ago, less than 25% of all prems survived. TODAY, however, thanks to the marvels of medicine and technology – collectively, 90% of all prems survive.

The chances of a Prem baby surviving outside the Mother's womb is influenced by a huge number of factors, but mostly depends on the degree of maturity of the baby's organs, because this affects such things like whether the baby is able to even BREATHE, whether the baby's fragile SKIN can hold in vital fluids, and whether the baby's BRAIN can handle the medical treatment necessary to keep the baby alive and all the early sensory stimulation.

Just think back to reading and learning about each stage of your pregnancy (like I did), the information supplied by websites or birthing books as to how your baby is growing week by week inside you, and imagine that time cut short way before all the important major 'groundwork' and internal 'plumbing 'is complete... And then that baby being forced out into a world it's not yet meant to be in, and quite literally, not ready for.

Even though there is now a 90% survival rate of Prems across the board, there are researched survival rate figures for EACH gestation, which has a sliding scale from each end.

For example: a baby born at 22 weeks only has between a 2%–15% chance of survival,

Whereas a baby born at 36 weeks has a 95%–100% chance of survival.

And it is a researched FACT, and interesting to know; that MALE Prems are slightly less matured and have a slightly HIGHER risk of mortality than females.

Not surprisingly, the more prematurely born the baby, the greater the severity of medical issues. For example, some IMMEDIATE complications a Prem baby faces after birth is:

- HYPOGLYCAEMIA (especially if S.G.A …… Small for Gestational Age) and HYPOCALCAEMIA >>>> both of which can cause convulsions that may produce long-term brain damage.

BRAIN HAEMORRAGES (bleeds on the brain) are common for Prem Babies, and can also have serious long-term effects.

HYPOTHERMIA (due to little or no subcutaneous fat layer under the skin), which *is* why Prem babies are housed inside closed humidicribs until they are 2kg in weight and can regulate and sustain their own body temperature.

And then you also have the all-important breathing issues due to immature lungs, which obviously a prem baby needs assistance with – but assistance of which can be a double-edged sword because, whilst this oxygen support is life giving, if it's given for too long or at too high a level, it can cause blindness; such a fine line with little room for error. It is widely documented that too much oxygen inside his humidicrib was the cause for Stevie Wonder's loss of eyesight – too much oxygen was directly linked to his diagnosis of R.O.P (Retinopathy of Prematurity), a condition of the eye that can cause total or partial blindness. R.O.P occurs when there is sudden introduction of oxygen to the system while the blood vessels of the eyes are still growing. In a Term born baby, these vessels have completed the process, but in a Premature born baby, the sudden interruption of this process puts the baby at greater risk of eyesight problems.

Regular eye testing each fortnight commences at the age of six weeks, and continues until visual evidence that the blood vessels have grown from the cornea to the outer rim of the eye. With the current way these tests are still performed in some hospitals, they are pretty ghastly to say the least, and was the only procedure I could not bring myself to be present at whilst being performed on my son. Any Premmie mum who has a baby born under 32 weeks of age will know exactly what I mean … these tests strike fear and horror into every parent. Special eye drops are administered to dilate the iris, and then metal eye retractors are used in conjunction with a steel rod probe, and hand drawn diagrams to map the progress of the blood vessels growing to the outer rim of the eye. To see it being performed looks quite barbaric, but it is a necessary evil. Early intervention means any abnormality is detected and corrected for a more positive future diagnosis.

In 2012, a major fundraiser was launched for Flinders Medical Centre Neonatal Unit (Adelaide, SA, Australia) by football legend Tony Modra after his wife Erica gave birth prematurely – and had to witness her baby go through the old school R.O.P procedure.

Later, in 2013, another inspiring Flinders Neonate Father, Rob Van Driel, started the now infamous 'Daddy's Little Legend Neonatal Appeal', and further enhanced what the Modra's had started.

A digital Retcam Machine costs AU$177,000 – and at the time of writing (late 2014), the monetary figure for this fundraising (for Flinders Neo) to purchase the revolutionary digital scanning Retcam machine was reached; meaning these eye tests will be performed in the very near future without such invasive procedures – which will be a welcome relief for parents and make the testing so much more efficient for the practitioners – and be much MUCH kinder on the babies.

A Prem baby is also more susceptible to a condition called NEC (Necrotising Enterocolitis) – where the immature bowels start to die off from either a bacterial infection or simply from being forced to function way too soon. This generally occurs within the first 3 weeks after birth, and can be fatal if not treated. NEC is treated according to its severity using the Bells Staging Criteria; either with antibiotics, extensive medical support or by surgery.

In addition to the IMMEDIATE above post – birthing complications surrounding Prems, there are also CATEGORY SPECIFIC health issues and outcomes, of which I won't go into in detail, because for each week of gestation, there is a list a mile long …

But the general 'blanket' long-term health issues that ALL prems are at risk of facing are:

SEVERE disabilities such as Cerebral Palsy, Intellectual impairment, blindness and deafness, with a combination of all of these occurring in about 10–25 % of all babies born EXTREMELY PRETERM (26–under 32 weeks).

Difficulties of a MILDER nature, such as SUBTLE forms of Cerebral Palsy and visual impairment, Chronic Lung Disease and Asthma, learning difficulties and behavioural problems such as A.D.D; occur in much higher numbers of around 50–60 % of ALL babies born preterm.

But no matter the gestation, it is vitally important to remember that EACH baby and situation is DIFFERENT … At NO time can any two Prems be compared to each other, Even those born OF the same gestation. It is paramount to remember that every Prem is unique, with their own individual host of health factors that ultimately determine the outcome of THEIR survival and long-term health. Just because you read about it, doesn't mean YOUR baby will have those same problems or outcomes.

As a matter of fact, I was contacted the week before my first book launch for BORN TOO SOON by a premmie mum who's baby was born at 24 weeks in February of 2013 – and he was given only a 20% chance of survival at birth, and she was told if he lived – he would have a 90% chance of having cerebral palsy.

But I am happy to say, he beat all those odds and is 100% healthy – just proof of how strong and determined is the fortitude of these little premmie miracles.

Every Neo Mum has a different story to tell, and each prem baby's health is individually intrinsic. And as traumatic as it may be for you to witness, never underestimate the sheer will to live that these little premmies have. As they say – it's not the size of the baby in the fight – but the size of the fight in the baby …

Here's an interesting fact!!! One of the greatest minds in history was born a Prem! He had intellectual development issues in the form of language delay and lack of speech fluency up until the age of nine – then he went on to become the renowned Genius and Physicist that we all know as … ALBERT EINSTIEN!! So take heart!!! Just because your baby was born a Prem, and may have to navigate a myriad of health issues and outcomes; does not mean they are not destined for Greater Things!!!!

Getting back to my Neonatal journey, suffice it to say, the birth I had planned was WAY off what it ended up being in reality. It was not the warm, fuzzy, bunny rug and nappy changing experience I had envisioned. The turn of events irreparably changed my whole life. I suffered in stoic silence for months after (with my state of mind) until I couldn't take it anymore and finally cracked and sought help.

It became apparent not long after our hospital stay that something wasn't right with me, but I stubbornly rejected the idea that there was something wrong, because I had always been such a strong-willed and strong-minded person.

How could someone like ME – who had (had) the nickname "REX" at work because I was tenacious and up front – be reduced to a slobbering, teary mess every five minutes? I felt like I'd had the life sucked out of me. I felt like an empty husk.

But if I'm totally honest – a more truthful and terrifying reason I stayed silent about how I was feeling for so long was out of fear – I didn't want to put myself on anyone's radar and have them take my baby from me. An ignorant and unfounded fear, but at the time it was very real. I already felt like I'd had my baby taken off me once – I didn't want that to happen again. By hell, I vowed to suck it up and soldier on.

Also, the long-term effects that our Prem Journey had on my life post Neo spilled over and impacted on everything I did, and HOW I did them – and I would have to say, it was in a somewhat malignant and negative way. Some of you may be able to identify with some of my behaviour, because I'm almost certain I'm not the only Neo Mum to have been affected in this way.

And after our whole Neo experience, just the mere thought of going out in public with *my* precious baby was so suffocating; that I unwittingly subjected myself to a self-imposed house arrest, and also deterred people from visiting.

On the one hand, I was so lonely and wanted – NEEDED – comfort, but I was so scared of my baby falling ill and ending up back in hospital. Going back to that cold, clinical environment was not a place I wanted to re-visit anytime soon. I saw germs on everything, everywhere. In my mind's eye, I could literally SEE the germs marching off of a surface and onto my baby and into his nose and mouth. I wouldn't even touch my son MYSELF until I had doused my hands in antibacterial gel, like as is the hygiene protocol in the Neo. I was terrified of germs to the extreme.

I became ultra-paranoid and would literally have a panic attack if someone said they were coming to visit.

But I will elaborate more on this subject towards the end; after you have read where I had BEEN, in order to appreciate where I ended UP, and the correlation between the two.

But one of the MOST debilitating factors – for ME – was the fact I had no control over what was happening. Anyone who knows me well KNOWS that in order for me to function, I have to be in control. I have the lovely misfortune of suffering from low self-esteem and low self-confidence, so to counter act that I like to be ultra-organised and in control of any situation. Not as in to dominate, but more as in to regulate.

I like continuity. I like routine. I like knowing exactly what I'm doing, how I plan to do it, and how long it's going to take. I left school at fifteen because I had secured myself a four-year Indentured Apprenticeship. I was in control of that. I left home at sixteen because I had a full-time job and could support myself. I was in control of that. When we married, we paid for absolutely everything ourselves – so I could be in control of every little detail to have the wedding of my dreams.

When we bought our house, it was as a direct result of decisions we had made from having distinct five-year plan goals to follow that we had set out for ourselves.

But when I gave birth prematurely, THAT was not something I had ANY control over, nor the events that followed as a direct result of it. And this is one factor that affected me greatly. Hell, I didn't even go to workplace staff shows and get drunk – because being drunk would mean I wasn't in control of not only my sobriety, but of my BEING. So to suddenly have my carefully thought out birth plans totally thwarted, and my expectations of new motherhood totally obliterated – you can maybe feel a tiny glimpse of just how totally bereft I felt. I lived on a knife edge for a bit over three months, and then some; as extenuating circumstances took hold. As well as having to deal with the heartache and fears of a premature birth, I also felt like I had lost who I was, due to having no control over my situation.

It's like floating away from earth, and feeling all gravity slipping away; fully aware of the choke hold it has on you but being powerless to stop it due to having nothing to grasp onto to keep you grounded ... the following sentiment is true, that you don't need water to feel like you are drowning.

MY NEO STORY is as follows ... which will explain how I believe I became more at risk of suffering Postnatal Depression, and hopefully it will liberate some Mums out there fighting their own struggle.

Because I want you all to know, in regards to both Premature Birth and Postnatal Depression – I cannot re-iterate it enough – YOU ARE NOT ALONE. The veritable landmine of emotions you experience are constant and unrelenting, and I do believe that these are universal feelings regardless of each individual situation. And I *know* that sometimes, even in your darkest hour, you are not looking for any specific advice or guidance – but simply an ear to hear you out; for someone to act as a sounding board to get it all off your chest, and for you to be understood and offered empathy, instead of being maligned and judged.

CHAPTER THREE

It was a week after we had celebrated our 15th Wedding anniversary when I found out I was pregnant with our first child. We had been trying for twelve months, but with each month that passed, I was beginning to think we had left our run too late. I was thirty-seven.

I had been on the contraceptive pill since I was fifteen. I was starting to think I had ruined my insides and my chances to conceive. Every barren month that went by took away just that little bit more of my aspirations to become a mother.

So seeing that second line show up on the test strip was a dream come true. I almost didn't believe it, so I did three more tests at various times of the day over the next two days; using all manner of test kits available; from the cheap supermarket jobs to the expensive chemist ones that pinpoint exactly how far along you were pregnant. They were all positive.

The wait to see my doctor to officially confirm my pregnancy took forever – even though it was only four days later. From the moment I took the pregnancy test, to the time I saw my doctor, I felt like I was holding my breath. I was so paranoid in that time (that I had to wait to see the doctor) that I would miscarry; that I tried not to cough, sneeze or even go to the toilet for number twos unless I absolutely HAD to!! I am a non-smoker, and I immediately went off caffeine, fizzy drinks and alcohol (not that I was a drinker, anyway).

I even stopped eating any type of take-away food. As a chef, I was ever conscious of food poisoning. If I didn't prepare it with my own hands, I didn't eat it. I followed the recommendations for steering clear of soft cheeses, shellfish, and mercury laden pelagic fish. I wanted to be as healthy as I could possibly be for the life I was now growing inside me.

Seeing that little flickering blip on the screen for the first time was surreal. I was a Mum! It changed my whole way of thinking. I started charting my future movements around all my scheduled Doctor's appointments; waiting in anticipation for each date to arrive, with every visit being just one more hurdle jumped. It was all I could think about.

My baby's development and wellbeing consumed my every thought, every day.

First was the dreaded Nuchal Translucency Test (Down Syndrome Test). The doctor I was seeing told me I was at a higher risk due to my age; 1 in 250 odds. So that was an anxious wait.

Then there was the twenty-week Morphology Scan. I invited my dad to that one, as there was no such thing as Ultrasounds back when my mum was pregnant with me; and I wanted to share this exciting venture with him – given that my baby was to be his first grandson.

My pregnancy, on the whole, was pretty much straight forward with no real hiccups to speak of. All my tests and scans came back clear and normal, but I had the most awful morning sickness up until week seventeen. Boy was I sick; all day, every day.

Some days I couldn't even get out of bed. It intrigues me WHY they call it Morning Sickness, when it can be any – and is often, every hour, day and night...

I also had bouts of real, sometimes severe stomach tenderness around my navel, which I had checked (up at the hospital) a couple of times, but I was told it was torn abdominal muscles and nothing to worry about – and it was suggested I wear a pregnancy brace which helps to hold up the weight of the "bump". I bought one from the Chemist, and it did make a difference.

Being my first pregnancy, I diligently enrolled in Antenatal Classes, which began for me at week twenty-four. In the next few weeks that followed we learnt that labour could potentially take DAYS to progress through all the stages (groan!), delivery was a given (have to finish what was started!) – and that the all-important skin-to-skin contact between mother and baby was done immediately after birth, with the baby being placed on the mother's bare chest as soon as it was born. That bit was talked about often. It was made to sound like it was a rite of passage. I was looking forward to that part the most, to finally meet my little one in the flesh instead of just being ringside at the football match being held inside my belly!! I had my Birth Plan all worked out. I knew what I DID and DID NOT want in the way of pain relief. Preferably, I wanted nothing that involved a needle, as I had a needle phobia. Certainly, I DID NOT want an epidural!!! The epidural demonstration in our Antenatal class had left me physically ill, but it also prompted me to start to wonder – how bad WAS labour pain, exactly – if one of the pain relievers was akin to getting knitting needles and fishing wire inserted between your vertebrae??

MY labour, of course, in my fantastical world, would not be too long; and there would be no need for medical intervention at the time of crowning and birth (i.e.: forceps, suction, episiotomy). I had started dreaming of that much talked about first skin-to-skin contact with my baby as it left my womb and we met each other visually for the first time. To gaze upon the face of the little life we had created. I was already preoccupied about what the colour of his hair would be, and the colour of his eyes. Would he be tall like his daddy? Would he have "piano fingers", or stumpy fat ones like his mummy? What sort of personality would he have? Would he be popular and have lots of friends? Or would he be like his mummy – a nerd and an introvert? What would his voice sound like? Or the sound of his laughter?

Photos would be taken of the first cuddles, first bath, first feed. I would have many visitors offering their well-wishes and wanting to meet our new arrival. Flowers. Hugs all round. I would be home in a couple of days. Someone might even make us a casserole or two once we were home. I had it all neatly planned, and I was anticipating my baby's due date with intoxicating excitement.

But at 4am on the 13th February, 2013; at 28+4 weeks gestation; my naïve little world collapsed. I was woken by what suspiciously felt like period pain, that would start out mild and build up to a crescendo before subsiding, then starting all over again shortly after. I remember laying there confused and wondering what had woken me up, and then I would feel it all over again; like a wave.

I knew this was not good, not at this early stage of gestation. And my pyjamas were wet. At first I thought I had lost control with the pressure of bubs on my bladder. But it didn't smell like urine. It smelt weirdly odd. Ever so faintly like chlorine. I knew that smell from years of breeding dogs and assisting with their whelps. I didn't want to believe or admit it, but I instinctively knew that (that) smell was amniotic fluid.

I rang the hospital, and the midwife told me to come up immediately. My husband had started to get dressed to drive me, but I reminded him that I was only twenty-eight weeks gone and still had three months (twelve weeks) to go yet before my due date; so instead of BOTH of us losing sleep, I would drive myself to the hospital. I tried to rationalise that it was a false alarm and that I would be back as soon as they had given me the all clear. I told him I would be back in time to cook his breakfast and see him off to work.

The drive to the hospital is only about eight minutes away from where we live, but it took me a little longer as I had to pull over twice for what I then knew, were definite *real* contractions. It finally dawned on me that my baby and I were in trouble.

At the hospital, I was examined and told I was being admitted. It was confirmed that I WAS INDEED in labour and that my waters had broken, but I wasn't dilated as yet.

I was given two doses of Celestone to try and stop the labour progressing, or to at least try and slow it down so that I could be transferred to Adelaide with my baby still "in-utero". It didn't work. The pain kept coming in waves. They were getting stronger and closer together. Then the phone calls began.

Medstar had already been notified and the RFDS was already on its way.

I called my husband and told him to come up straight away. I rang my sister, who had been coming to Antenatal classes with me and was my Birth Partner. She in turn rang my parents, who are divorced but both were living in Millicent at the time and ¾ of an hour away. She also rang my boss and told him I wouldn't be returning to work. I had still had seven weeks of work left before I was due for five weeks off before my due date.

I can still remember the immense guilt I felt and feeling like I had let my boss and co-workers down. So much was left unfinished, and I felt so at odds because I'm the type of person who likes everything in its place and organised.

I was given steroid injections to help with my baby's immature lungs, and put on a magnesium drip to help with his brain. The magnesium drip was especially nasty – it made me feel like my whole body was about to spontaneously combust. The GP on shift was paged, and a paediatrician was called to be on hand also.

My parents arrived, and as my dad is devoutly religious, I asked him to pray; to pray for the safe passage of my baby, and for his health. It was shortly after that, that I felt like I had to push, and when the midwife checked she found I was suddenly 9cm dilated.

All of the above was happening while I had my eyes clamped firmly closed.

I figured if I couldn't SEE what was happening, then maybe it wasn't. Pity my body didn't understand the correlation and co-operate... all I remember of my labour and birth was blackness. I was too scared to open my eyes.

At 8:44am, surrounded by my family with my husband holding onto my hand, *our baby* was born. A little boy, weighing 1350gm (2.98 pound) and the length of a 2ltr milk carton. He had good APGAR scores – 8 and 10 respectively. And he was breathing on his own when he came out into the world. We named him Aidan.

On the up-side, I had gotten PART of my Birth Plan: my labour was only just over four hours long from start to finish, and I had no pain relief or any medical intervention at time of birth. But that's where my dream birth ended.

Instead of being placed on my chest, my baby was whisked away to be prepared for Flight with the MEDSTAR team. I got to see him for the first time about an hour after I delivered him. I was stunned. In my mind, I had envisioned my baby would be wrapped in muslin with a beanie on and sucking on a dummy – instead I found him naked except for an over-sized nappy, on CPAP oxygen and hooked up to cardio monitoring. He was crying ever so softly that it sounded more like a kitten meowing; and when I touched his hand his tiny fingers grasped onto one of mine and held on surprisingly tight. But still I couldn't hold him.

I watched on as the MEDSTAR team took what seemed like copious amounts of blood, for which instead of a heel prick they actually had nicked his tiny foot open with a scalpel in order to get the volume of blood they needed. I was horrified that they would/could do such a thing to such a tiny baby!! And to MY baby!!!! I was outraged and sickened both at the same time.

They also gave him so many injections – drugs to stabilise him for flight; and I remember questioning them at the time to make sure they had the correct dose for his tiny little body. I watched on in disbelief as all this was happening, and I was powerless to stop it. I was terrified for him.

We were both flown by RFDS to Flinders Medical Centre in Adelaide, and I remember feeling like I was in a metal coffin. I was strapped to the gurney which was so close to the roof of the plane. I had to keep my eyes shut the entire trip and concentrate on my breathing so I wouldn't have a panic attack or feel claustrophobic. I could hear the MEDSTAR midwife, nurse and doctor on board constantly commenting on the beeps and dings of the humidicrib Aidan was in. At one stage the midwife got up to get a beanie for Aidan because apparently he was getting cold. He was still naked except for a nappy. The one dominating thought going through my mind the whole flight over to Adelaide was the comment made by one of the attending midwives at my son's birth a couple hours after I had delivered him. In the ensuing race to get Aidan prepared for emergency retrieval, she blithely said to me in passing – "I thought I would be consoling you right now." Up until that point, I had been deliberately naive. I hadn't allowed myself to think of any alternative negative outcome. I was well aware he was born too early; but he was alive, and he was breathing – and I was hanging onto that fact with every fibre of my being. But she had now put new horrors in my head with just that one casual remark, and I silently prayed that he would hang in there until we got to Flinders, where the Perinatal Specialists and revered Neonatologists were.

When we landed, once again my precious baby and I were separated. We were transported to Flinders Hospital in separate ambulances. The MT in the back of the ambulance with me commented how her partner (who was driving) was "keeping up" with the Ambulance in front so I "wasn't too far away from my baby". I know she meant well and was trying to comfort me, but all I could think of was: too late.

When we pulled up, the gurney I was on was wheeled in behind Aidan's through Admissions and Emergency, and for a brief minute they put us side by side so I could see him again, but then Aidan was briskly wheeled away and taken to the

Neonatal Unit while I was taken up to the Maternity Ward. It was another few hours before I was allowed to go and see him, and lying in my hospital room I felt desolate, grieved and scared. My mind was in torment. What were they doing to my son? How was he?? WHERE was he???

I didn't even have any clothes to change into. I couldn't even do my hair or brush my teeth. My Husband had rushed home after I had given birth to throw together a hospital bag for me, but I wasn't allowed to take it on the RFDS due to storage restrictions. My sister and mum were travelling up by car and were bringing it with them, but they wouldn't be there until the next day. All I had with me were the clothes on my back that I had driven up to the hospital in (in) the wee hours of the morning, my mobile phone, and some money my husband had thrust at me. I felt uncharacteristically dirty. It seemed even my own personal hygiene was now out of my control. I was beyond the point of caring what I looked like, but I desperately wanted to physically wash away the remnants of my ordeal from the last few hours.

I felt numb. I could barely comprehend the fact that I had indeed given birth hours earlier. It didn't seem real. It had all happened so fast.

A nurse went and rustled up some food and a drink for me, and showed me the little kitchenette down the corridor – for if I wanted a hot tea or coffee. She told me she would be back later to take me to see Aidan. I was left by myself with just my thoughts and fears. I had never felt more alone in my life. I was wracked with guilt and sick with worry for my tiny baby. I tried, but I couldn't cry. The tears just wouldn't come. I sat in my hospital room for the next few hours, just staring blindly out the window at the rooftops of other wards, wondering what they were doing to my baby and if he was okay. I wanted answers, a REASON for why this had happened to me – and my baby - but no-one could give me any. There WAS no reason.

I was so unprepared for what I was confronted with when a nurse finally took me down to the NeoNatal Unit (NNU).

At no time during our Antenatal classes were we told of what to expect if our babies were born premature. All we were told was – if you give birth before thirty-four weeks, you go to Adelaide. That was it.

Sure, I had vague flashbacks of seeing something like this on TV, but to actually see it for yourself, and involving your own baby … I was distraught and beside myself.

After being swiped in through the security doors I was taken through the Unit, past dozens of plastic bubbles and monitors that each housed a tiny baby inside; until we stopped at the one that contained Aidan.

He was still on CPAP oxygen, which covered most of his face, and now also had surgical central lines directly into his belly button, drips in both arms, a tube down his throat and a myriad of cords and leads hooked up to the various machines beside his bubble. He was naked except for a nappy that was way too big. He had bruises on his head, face and arms from delivery trauma, and I noticed his skin was so fragile and thin that you could see the veins underneath like a road map. My first thought was *what if he gets tangled in all those cords?* There were so many of them, with clips and clamps and tags they had written on. Irrationally, I wondered how the babies didn't suffocate inside their plastic 'boxes' – because the isolettes are sealed top to bottom to keep the heat in and the germs out. Pretty obvious, when you could barely see your baby's face underneath the contraption that was giving him oxygen – but when I was first introduced to the visual hard reality of the Neo, my mind was taking in so much at once that I was confused. I was looking without really seeing.

I was heartbroken and felt a suffocating despair. How could this have happened?

And WHY?? He was meant to still be INSIDE me, not inside this plastic womb! He didn't deserve this. And I STILL hadn't had my first cuddle. I felt ripped off. I had given birth but was being denied the process of being a real mum. At the most, I could only touch him through the portholes of his humidicrib.

Coming to terms with the fact my body had failed him and that he would now be "artificially grown" inside this sterile sea of technology and looked after 24/7 by a rotation of nurses was rudely humbling. All I could do was sit beside his bubble and watch him breathe. I visited him periodically throughout the night, as there was no way I could sleep. Each time I left the Maternity ward I had to fill in and sign the chart at the front counter saying what time I had left, where I was going, and what time I would be back. I left that last bit open, as I couldn't put a time limit on how long I would be. All I wanted was to be close to my son; to see him and watch over him, and silently scream inside. I apologised to him over and over. This was not the way it was meant to have been, for either of us, but especially for him.

I fondly remember his assigned NICU nurse took a photo of him for me the very first night, and printed it off on a camera dock – so I could have him 'with' me at all times. It was a clear shot of his delicate little face, and I could instantly see he had his father's indignant chin, clearly visible below the nasal prongs.

She also gently explained that by gazing at his photo whilst expressing my milk, it would help with 'let down' and volume. When I wasn't physically by his side, I would sit in my hospital room just staring at this photo for hours.

His beautiful little face was the last thing I would see before going to sleep at night, and the first thing I saw when I woke. That one thoughtful gesture of a simple photo taken by his Neo nurse is what got me through the first few days after my son's early arrival, and it helped me adjust to us being separated. It was my visual connection, and it was unnervingly powerful the emotions it would evoke by just looking at it. It's the little things like this that the Neo Staff do, that makes them so good at their jobs. They are so intuitive and empathic. To anyone else, the meaning of a simple photo would be overlooked. But to a struggling new Neo Mum, that photo meant everything and was priceless. These nurses truly are the heart and soul of the NICU. They seem to know what you need before you yourself even know it.

The next day I crashed emotionally.

I was sitting on the toilet in my hospital room when it happened. It hit me like a lightning bolt, and I felt frazzled to the core. I felt like I was being strangled, like I couldn't breathe. I couldn't stop the tears. I missed my husband. I missed the familiarity of my home. I missed my dogs. I missed my family. I missed work.

But most of all, I missed not being pregnant anymore. On more than one occasion, I was SURE I could still feel my baby kicking inside me, and then reality checked in to remind me that he was in fact, downstairs, inside his plastic bubble, being closely watched by his nurse. Being cared for by someone other than me, his mother. I felt inadequate. I was angry. No one had any answers as to why. I might have accepted it a bit better had I been given a reason as to WHY my body had decided it couldn't carry my baby any further. I had been fit and healthy and done all the right things. All I was told was – Probable Sepsis, nothing definitive. I felt incredibly guilty. Aidan deserved much better than this.

I took my sister and mum down to see Aidan when they arrived later that morning, and after they left I had a much needed shower and sleep; before continuing my regular trips downstairs to visit my baby. Later that night I was shown by a nurse how to hand express my milk, which I was to collect in a syringe and take down to the NNU so they could give it to Aidan through his feeding tube. My first effort yielded only a few drops. But as it was colostrum, I was told every single drop counted. So I diligently set to task occupying myself in my room by expressing every couple of hours.

The next try I got .2 of a ml. Then .5 of a ml. Then .7 – until I eventually expressed a full 1ml!! At last I had something to do that benefitted Aidan.

Something only I could do for him as his Mummy.

CHAPTER FOUR

Once I was discharged as a patient from hospital, I was allocated one of the flats (at the back of the hospital) that used to be the old nurses quarters, specifically refurbished and reserved for Neo Mum's more than 100km from home. There are three flats reserved for the Neo, with three bedrooms in each flat – so at any one time, they can accommodate nine Neo mums. Each bedroom has two beds, and you are allowed to have your partner or a support person stay with you also. Each bedroom is private and lockable. You share the rest of the flat; the bathroom, toilet, lounge and kitchen. Everything except food is provided. Even a cleaner comes in once a week. The flat has all the comforts of home. Fully self-contained, from the large screen TV, to the electric wok in the cupboard.

I cannot begin to express my gratitude for having been housed in one of those flats.

I could never have afforded to rent any accommodation for the length of time Aidan was a patient in the Neo. Had it not been for those emergency flats, I probably would have had to leave Aidan in Adelaide and come home. That would have literally killed me, I think; to be THAT far away from him for THAT length of time. But as fate would have it (or faith, as I believe), I had somewhere to sleep and it was conveniently only about an eight minute leisurely walk away from where Aidan was. And I now also had a security tag so I could swipe myself into the NNU at any time of the day or night, 24/7.

I reluctantly went home with my sister and mum back to Mount Gambier that weekend, three days after giving birth and arriving in Adelaide; so I could get my car, some more clothes, some food for the flat and also so my dad could come back and stay with me in the flat for moral support and company.

Leaving Aidan in the hospital to go home for twenty-four hours was the hardest thing I ever had to do. It was like my heart was being squeezed. I was sobbing as we left; it hurt so unbelievably much to leave him. I said my goodbyes half a dozen times, leaving his crib side each time and getting to the outer doors of the NNU, but then hurrying back to him for one last look or touch. I know the nurses could do more for him than I could at this point, but it just felt WRONG leaving him. He was MY baby. I should be sitting next to him, watching over him. Not 500 odd kilometres away! And what if something happened to him while I was gone, and I wasn't there for him?

But then, I also needed to see my husband too; to be held in his arms and be told it would all be okay; to process it all with him. To try and make some sort of sense of what had happened. I was one entity that needed to be in two places at once, but could only be in one. That's what also made it so hard to accept. We were now a family and should all be together! But my husband couldn't be with me in Adelaide as he had work commitments and had to look after our animals and the house. At a time when we should have been rejoicing and celebrating, we were separated. We hadn't even discussed the events surrounding Aidan's birth yet. I had no idea of the impact this had all had on him. But I'm sure he was just as traumatised from it. And it would have been just as hard on him, being so far away and not knowing from one hour to the next how his son was doing; waiting on tender hooks for each text message update from me. I phoned the Neo Unit's Dedicated Parent Line every hour from home to speak directly to his personal nurse and check on Aidan, and even though I was only gone for one day, it felt like forever. I couldn't relax while I was at home, because I was always thinking of the absence of my baby. Then, when it was time to leave home and go back to Adelaide, I didn't want to go. I cried and cried.

I needed my husband, and the familiarity of my own home. The Neonatal Ward scared me; it was foreign, high tech, impersonal, clinical and so, so far from home.

I didn't want to go back there; yet I DID want to, because that's where my baby was, and ultimately where I wanted to be. I was torn.

Once I got back to Flinders, my whole world revolved around and inside the NNU.

I spent every day from dawn till dusk beside Aidan's humidicrib. I only went back to the flat periodically to shower, eat and sleep. It was the middle of summer, and the days were hot and sticky, and the short walk to and from the flat half a dozen times a day was an effort in itself in the heat. Plus, the NNU is kept at a constant warm temperature for the babies. I always felt like I'd had a shower and dressed while still wet. But luckily, the flats had air-conditioning. What a godsend.

I felt a bit bad for my dad, as he was only allowed to visit Aidan during the stipulated visiting hours – so while I was down with my baby, my dad was left alone in the flat to amuse himself. But I appreciated his sacrifice for being up there with me more than he will ever know; it was comforting to have another person to go "home" to after a tense and draining day sitting by Aidan's crib. And I especially liked the fact that before we went to bed each night, my dad would give me a hug.

That was extra special; sort of like a band-aid for all of my hurt.

After that first week, I took another quick trip back to Mount Gambier to drop my dad off, pay some bills, see my husband for all of twenty-four hours and then back to Adelaide; this time with my mum coming back to stay with me to keep me company.

But the first night she was there was very trying. I had developed a blood clot in my leg just behind the knee that morning; and upon arriving back in Adelaide after a five-hour drive, I showed it to the Neo Ward doctors; and they told me to go down to Accident and Emergency and have it examined ASAP – so we spent another five long hours down there WAITING for my turn to be seen …time I resented I wasn't spending with Aidan. I hadn't seen him for a bit over twenty-four hours. I was distressed because the time wasted in the waiting room was time I was not beside his crib; plus I was hungry, tired; and my clot was hot, throbbing and painful. The doctor I finally saw was impressed with the size of the clot – by now you could cup it in the palm of your hand. But she assured me it wasn't a venous (DVT) clot, but a varicose clot.

The former is the dangerous one, the latter not so much. She also sent me for an ultrasound on it the next day just to make sure of her diagnosis. It was well after 2am by the time I had been seen and we could go back to the flat. We had been travelling all day and hadn't eaten tea due to waiting in the A & E all night. I wanted to go and see Aidan, but I was exhausted. After some toast, a short sleep and a shower, I was back at Aidan's side before the sun had even come up. My daily crib side vigils continued, and mum would stay in the flat until visiting hours.

Looking back now, on reflection, I think this was the time when my mum and I started to repair our mother-daughter relationship. Until I had fallen pregnant, we had been estranged for a few many years. The birth of my son had begun to heal the rift.

At least SOMETHING good had come out of our bad situation. My mum was back in my life. And I openly admit – I needed her now, more than ever.

Yet another quick twenty-four-hour trip back to Mount Gambier after mum's one-week stay with me, with my dad returning with me again for another week. We resumed our former routine, and when I took dad home after that week, he bought me a laptop – to keep me occupied and amused when I wasn't with Aidan. Because now, after the first three weeks of having company in the flat with me, I returned there and was alone.

It was just me and my daily treks to and from the Neo, with nothing but my mobile phone for contact with the outside world. I took and sent multiple photos of Aidan daily (on my phone) and sent them to my husband for updates; and the daily text messages with my hubby and family was about the extent of my company and support outside the walls of the Neo. But my new laptop kept me in the loop also, and gave me something to do at night when I couldn't sleep. Facebook, which I'd never been too keen on, became my new best friend.

For the first six weeks, I had the flat to myself; with the exception of a couple of new Neo mums spending a few nights with me also. Then circumstance had it that I was swapped from that flat to another flat that already had two other resident mums – long-term Neo mum's like myself. Coming back to the flat late at night and having other people there was comforting. We would sit in the lounge room and discuss our days; the highs and lows, the tears and joys. We could be frank with each other, lay ourselves bare – we were all going through the same nightmare. It wasn't long before I felt like I had known these ladies forever. Just their mere presence made it bearable.

But behind the closed door of my bedroom each night, I cried myself to sleep – for the unfairness and injustice of it all. For the sorrow and guilt I felt. For the pain and suffering Aidan was being forced to endure daily. I hoped and prayed that he wouldn't remember any of this.

I FINALLY GOT MY FIRST CUDDLE when Aidan was 5 days old; when the central umbilical lines were removed. It was after I had returned from my first trip back from Mount Gambier from collecting my dad. It was the single most, joyous feeling in the world!! Even though I was scared to death of holding him because he was so tiny and had so many wires attached to him, it is a moment I will never forget. I was acutely aware that he didn't have that fresh intoxicating new baby smell – just one more thing I was ripped off of. My baby smelt clinical, like the sanitising gel that is spread around the Neonatal Unit on every bench and wall like the interior designer had OCD. But once I had him in my arms, I didn't want to give him back. To feel this tiny little human wriggling every so often on my bare chest was surreal.

After that first initial cuddle, I was allowed to have a daily cuddle with him; with the nurse getting him out of his bubble for me each time due to all his cords etc. They made it look so easy, deftly handling him to get him in and out, or changing his position in his nest; all the while moving his many cords in unison with the prose of a maestro.

I would go down before early morning shift change when it was nice and quiet so I could enjoy it all the more. But even a simple cuddle wasn't without risk. If I didn't hold him right, with his head and neck at just the right angle, his respiratory monitor would go off because his air supply was compromised. Everything was so nerve-racking. It was hard to have a special bonding moment when the machines were constantly beeping and the nurse had to keep coming to check on him and reposition him on my chest; or check his oxygen nasal probes or his cardio leads. A lot of times, our cuddles would have to be cut short and Aidan put back in his bubble because it was all just too over-stimulating for him, and his little body couldn't handle it. In these times, I just had to make do with holding his little hand through the isolette porthole.

I gradually learnt what the beeps and dings and alarms of the many machines meant, and I picked up the overload of medical lingo pretty quick. In the beginning, all of this overwhelmed me and I would sit with tears in my eyes, listening to the alarms going off and watching the nurses attending to Aidan, and mentally torturing myself as to what was happening. Learning how to properly read the machine's numbers and diagnostics made it easier to accept what was happening and understand. I'm sure Aidan's nurses were sick of me, as I was always asking questions and checking what they were doing to him and why. I made it my business to know all that was being done to him. But they were always more than happy to explain, and were friendly about it – consummate professionals. They went out of their way to give me reassurance. From day one, I was witness to all of Aidan's daily blood tests and the various procedures performed on him. I watched on anxiously as he had daily multiple Bradycardias, Apneas and Desats. I was present for his cranial ultrasounds and lung X-rays. I sat with him through his blood transfusions. As hard as it was to see my tiny baby go through it all, I didn't want him to go through it alone. It was because of me that he was in this predicament to start with, so the least I could do was be there for him.

I remember being allowed to change his nappy for the first time. Every procedure done to him was done through the portholes of his bubble. So it was like doing it with your opposite hand and with the other one tied behind your back – and like reaching around a fish tank; it was so foreign and tricky and not a lot of room to move in, and on top of it all you had to juggle all that with all of his leads and cords in the way! But somehow, I managed. It was a case of having to.

And I remember being beside myself with nervous excitement when I got to feed him through his feeding tube for the first time. Milk is delivered via a syringe that fits just perfectly to the stopper on the end of the tube; so you pull back the plunger on the syringe, unscrew the cap on the tube, twist in the syringe end and pull the plunger completely out; then hold the syringe up slightly for gravity to suck the milk down the feed tube into his tummy. Once the syringe is empty, carefully pop the plunger back in the end of the syringe, twist it off and plug the cap back on the end of the feed tube. This is called a Bolus feed, or Drop feed or Gravity feed. All are one and the same.

I got to be so excited to be able to do this small thing every hour for my baby. Not conventional feeding, but being fed none the less with MY milk, by MY hand. It started out being 1ml every hour and gradually rising – subject to his little body being able to cope with the increased volume. I remember my dad saying, "But how can he survive on just 1ml per hour?" But he was also hooked up to intravenous Lipids and PNS (Parenteral Nutrition Solution), set to flow at a certain volume for his body weight.

The nurses would do an hourly aspirate; whereby they use a syringe to suck the previous milk feed BACK OUT of his stomach via the feeding tube, to see how much of it has been digested. If the aspiration is more than 10% of the previous feed, it is syringed back in and the next scheduled feed held off. Or, if it's not looking digested (like curdled milk) or contains bile (tainted green), the next feed is also held back.

More than a few times this happened, and quite often Aidan had to be switched to being fed by Perfuser machine – where the milk is continuously administered slowly over the hour, instead of it being delivered in one hit, every hour. Being fed by Perfuser is a step backwards. The aim (in the long-term) is to get the babies fed by Bolus feeds every four hours. But it's a long process.

I got to bath him for the first time when he was seven weeks old, when he had graduated from his humidicrib into an open crib. The babies stay in their humidicribs until they are 2kg and over; when they can regulate and maintain their own body heat. Before that, it was just sponge baths through the portholes of his bubble. Being attached to the cardio machines with all the leads meant the bath was wheeled to his crib side and bathed there. But giving him that first real bath was exhilarating!!

Another bonus when he came out of the humidicrib into an open crib was that I was *able* to hold him more whenever I wanted (within reason) – and not have to ASK permission every time and have to get the nurse to get him out for me. It was a bit of freedom; a bit of normality. It was starting to feel like he WAS my baby, after all.

I took immense pleasure in doing even the most mundane things for him, like change a nappy or do his Cares. But leaving him every night in the NNU to go back to the flat was still beyond painful. Any new mum can relate how it would feel, going home empty handed. Right from the moment you discover you are pregnant, you bond with your baby. Then after that, all you want is to have your baby with you. Every night I left the NNU, I felt like I was missing a vital part of me – which I literally was.

By now I had stopped going back to the flat during the day – I left before the sun rose each morning and I had security drive me back well after midnight each night. Initially, I walked myself back to the flat each night for the first several weeks – the path was well lit, and I didn't see a problem with it. But the nurses got wind of it, and told me it wasn't safe and that there had been a few "incidents" in the past; which is when I started going down to the Security office for my escorts back. I hated having to ask them for a lift back to the flats each night – I felt like I was imposing and putting them out. I felt guilty each and every night that I went down to their office in the twilight hours and knocked on their window to ask for a lift, knowing the flats were just a couple of clicks down the road and I was interrupting their down time. But by the same token, I also needed to think of my safety – because my *son* needed me.

CHAPTER FIVE

For a total of 91 days (13 weeks), I practically lived inside the NNU. After a while, I ate all my meals in the Parent Room or Visiting Lounge. I would pack my breakfast, lunch and tea in my backpack each morning before I left the flat. I existed on microwave porridge sachets, Sunrice microwave ready meals, Suimin noodle cups and slices of Woolworths Select apple cinnamon cake. And coffee.* Lots and lots of coffee. The hospital Iced Coffee vending machines certainly got a work out from me...

I was present every morning as the Ward Doctors and a Paediatric Consultant did their rounds. They came around daily, with their entourage of medical students and fellows, the Neonate Unit Senior and at least one of the daily assigned nurses to the babies in each bay, to painstakingly assess each and every baby, and progress is discussed, or lack of it if that was the case, and decisions are made about oxygen requirements, milk volume, tests to be carried out and medications needing to be given for that day. I would sit and wait for these daily consults with bated breath, to see how my little baby was doing and chat to the Neonatal Specialist. I viewed them as Gods. I hung on their every word. I trusted them implicitly.

I expressed my milk every three hours, 24/7, for 13 weeks; either in the designated Expressing Room or beside Aidan's crib, going through the routine each time of putting one of

Aidan's computer generated ID stickers on the bottle and the date and time expressed, and then putting it in the milk fridge for collection by the milk nurse.

Right from when I started lactating and my milk had just come down, I felt like I *was* a dairy cow on a production line. It felt like I had only just expressed, and then was going through the whole routine yet again. I couldn't even sleep more than three hours overnight without having to express. On my trips back to Mt Gambier, I would have to stop and express at least once, sometimes twice. Everything I did had to be planned around my expressing times; it was like I was in servitude to my own *breasts*.

His nurses would tell me that Aidan knew when I was present next to his crib *because* his STATS would stabilise and he would be more restful. I took comfort in that. It was precisely this reason alone that I consciously and purposely wore the same perfumed body wash each and every day whilst my baby was in the Neo. It was the same fragrance as my signature perfume, but I was always worried if I actually wore my perfume that it may affect his breathing ability, so the subtle lingering scent of my body wash was the next best option.

I wanted for him to be able to distinguish ME from anyone else he came in contact with; to associate THAT fragrance with his mummy. Whether it WAS my scent, or the fact that he just instinctively KNEW me apart from the nurses, I was placated when the nurses would tell me that my mere presence had a calming and positive effect on my son.

I would read "The Cat in the Hat" to Aidan almost daily, and he seemed to like it. I bought it from the hospital gift shop a couple of days after we arrived there.

Even if he was asleep, I could see a subtle shift in his head towards me every so often, as though he were listening to my voice and my every word. I would tell him how his Daddy was going to teach him how to play football and cricket and how to catch a fish and use a slug gun when he was older. I would also softly sing or hum *Amazing Grace* or *Mockingbird* to him through the portholes of his humidicrib, or when we were having our daily cuddles.

I had also gotten quite adept by this time to power sleeping upright on the stool next to Aidan's crib; or having a nap on the armchair out in the Visiting Lounge. More than a few times, when I was in the breastfeeding chair having a cuddle with Aidan, I dozed off with him on my chest. Lucky there are multiple nurses around, and they kept an eagle eye on me so I didn't drop him. It was hard NOT to doze off when I had him on my chest – it's such a warm, loving, shut-the-world-out kind of feeling and you just get caught up in the moment, breathing in unison with your baby and switching off to everything. You just shut your eyes to savour it and pretend it's just you and your baby and no-one else.

I decorated Aidan's crib with a few finger puppets that I bought down in the hospital gift shop. A giraffe (befittingly, the universal symbol of a premmie Unit), a chicken and an elephant, so that he had something to focus on when he turned his head from side to side, and to keep him company when I wasn't there. That was the absolute worst – knowing that when I left, apart from the nurses attending to his four- hourly cares, his allocated meds and his feeds; he was alone with no-one to cuddle him or keep him company.

I attended some of the workshops offered to the mums on the Neo Ward, and I sat in on the Baby Safety and Resuscitation course more than a few times.

On Sundays, if Aidan's feed times allowed, I would attend the hospital chapel service. The chaplain would say a special prayer for Aidan each time.

We graduated from ICU in week four, into the Special Care Unit (which is still located inside the NNU). That day was another milestone … it was the day he was able to wear CLOTHES for the first time!! His nurse took me to a cupboard and told me I could pick out some clothes to dress him in – I was like a kid in a candy store! Of course, the smallest that was there were size 00000, and still too big for my baby, but I picked out the cutest little bodysuit and lovingly dressed him in it nonetheless.

In the SCU, as Aidan made steady progress, we made our way down through the bays (there are four bays, with six babies and two nurses in each bay).

I was told that each bay shift is a step closer to the door – i.e. to going home.

After five weeks in SCU, in week nine, we were taken upstairs to the Satellite Nursery on the Maternity Ward. What they dub the "Fattening Farm". It's the last step in the Unit for premmie babies; and those who are no longer deemed high risk, are sent upstairs to 'chub up' before going home.

Except for going back down to the NNU for twenty-four hours for a blood transfusion, Aidan spent the next four weeks in the Satellite Nursery. I was in two minds as to whether I liked being up in the Satellite Nursery. Up there, there are eight babies to two nurses, so *less* one-on-one time for each baby. I always worried he would be left crying if I wasn't there with him while the nurses attended to all the other babies. Not that it would be intentional, but each baby has their own medications that need to be given at certain times, which always needs to be done by BOTH nurses; and they were all on different feed schedules, some by bottle and others by gastric tube. Not to mention nappy changes, clothing changes if a baby had bad reflux and vomited, crib bedding changes, scheduled weighs and tests to be carried out … Some shifts those poor nurses were run ragged!

And up there, it was less 'clinical' – something that made me very uneasy after spending nine weeks saturated in beeping monitors and alarms going off and copious amounts of Aquim gel. The nurses wouldn't even touch the pen on a baby's chart without using Aquim before and after. And the silence was deafening. Apart from the chorus of crying babies, the room was much too quiet. BUT – the Satellite Nursery had one whole wall that was a window – which meant natural

SUNSHINE in the room!! That alone gave a whole new ambience to the room. And, up there, you were allowed to wheel your baby in their crib out of the room to the lounge area just outside the door, and sit in the direct sunshine and watch all the traffic and pedestrians below on the street front. In ICU and SCU, there are no windows. It's all artificial light. If it weren't for the clocks on the walls, and the staff shift changes, you would never know the time of day.

You tend to lose all modesty and inhibitions while you are in the NNU. Flinders is a breastfeeding endorsed hospital, and it's a natural practice – so amidst the hub – bub of activity in the NNU, there are a lot of exposed breasts; either breast feeding or expressing milk – and I never once felt ashamed or embarrassed or viewed it as out of the ordinary. After all – the whole reason all of us mums were there was because of our babies. And babies need to be fed – simple as that.

Prem babies aren't naturally born with the suck, swallow, breathe reflex – it has to be learnt, so there is a lot of "breast" play and nipple sucks going on to help their progress. And if you need help or your baby has problems attaching, a midwife or speech pathologist comes to help. Even with so many foreign hands touching my breasts, I never once felt self-conscious, because it was all to benefit Aidan.

And that was all that mattered.

It took me a while, but eventually I had accepted that THIS was my lot in life, and I unknowingly allowed myself to become institutionalised to hospital procedure and politics. I had my security key card to let myself in and out of the Neo Unit. I came and went as a matter of course. The machines and alarms and constant activity that at first had terrified and overwhelmed me, eventually became white noise and the "norm" and oddly comforting. I had my perch next to my baby and I sat there; day in, day out, while the nurses bustled on around me. I became 'part of the furniture'.

For the most part, I was alone pretty much the whole time we were in Adelaide in Hospital. As already mentioned, my husband had (had) to stay in Mount Gambier due to work and home commitments. That in it bought a lot of questions and innuendo from my hospital assigned social worker, and made me very angry at times because not every case is clear cut black and white. Everybody's situation in the NNU is personal and unique – and you just have to do what works for YOU. Being separated from each other was an added heartache for both of us, but we thought it out logically and did what was best for US in OUR circumstance. We both agreed the short-term inconvenience was for a long-term gain, and despite how hard it was, we were okay with that. But because my social worker made me feel uncomfortable, I hid every time I saw her come into the NNU. Just so I wouldn't have to deal with her. Sometimes she caught up with me. Most times she didn't. She was a nice enough lady to talk to in passing, but her job description meant I always felt like she was dissecting every fibre of my being, and I didn't appreciate the supposition and conjecture, and I felt like she was just waiting for me to fall to pieces and pounce on me.

My sister and Mum had come up initially for a few days, then my dad stayed with me in weeks one and three, and Mum in week two. I don't think I could have survived those first few initial weeks without my parents' support. And my sister was my rock. Despite having three kids of her own, being in the middle of building a house and having a job; she made a special trip over and spent one weekend with me in the flat. And she kept me grounded with daily phone calls and text messages. My bosses' wife and their daughter were in Adelaide for an appointment, and also came to visit me and meet Aidan. My husband flew over one weekend in the sixth week to see his son for the second time since he was born.

It must have been hard on him, being separated from his wife and baby boy. My whole premature birth and post birthing experience was also not something he had been counting on, or even paid thought to. As a result of the calamity, immediately after Aidan was born, my husband couldn't bring himself to look at him, stating 'he didn't look real'.

But the paternal protectiveness he FELT despite the situation was VERY real – he kept a pacing vigil at the doorway of the room that the Medstar Team were prepping Aidan in before we were transferred, concern and worry etched all over his face for his preterm infant son, the fruit of his loins.

Now, even weeks later, the confronting reality of Aidan's early birth was clearly palpable, and though he didn't say much, the look in his eyes, and the expression on his face when he saw Aidan in his bubble, and one sentence spoken, said it all: "I can't believe we made him. He is tiny, but perfect; ten fingers, ten toes – and his Mummy's button nose."

I will remember those words forever. We sat quietly beside Aidan for a few hours, he listening while I explained my daily routine and the mechanics of the machines; and judging by the angst on his face and his wide eyes, I could see him taking in the enormity of the whole situation. Being physically there in the middle of it was so far removed to him just receiving regular text updates from me. He already knew how traumatic it was for me to be in there with our son day in, day out – but I don't think he REALLY appreciated the true extent until he himself was actually sitting in that austere environment.

Other than that, I had very few visitors. Only seven visits in ninety-one days. And most of them were from Paul's niece. My husband's sister also made a special trip to see us in hospital, despite her own health problems, but her trip was in vain because she was allowed to see only me, not Aidan. I felt particularly bad about that, because I know how hard it was for her to have made the three-hour round trip, but if you so much as have even a sniffle, you aren't allowed into the Neo Unit – obviously with good reason.

It was hard, especially when other mums had their partners with them, and a constant flow of well-wishers at visiting times. At these times, I usually sat tucked away in the corner of our bay station and occupied myself by either quietly talking to, or reading, to Aidan.

At night in the flat, at least twice a week, I would bake cupcakes and decorate them for the Neo nurses and ward doctors for morning tea. It was something to keep me occupied, and was also a small gesture of gratitude for everything they were doing for our baby. They seemed to like them – there were never any left at the end of the day.

I celebrated my 38th birthday, Easter and first Mothers' Day inside the NNU.

My kind fellow Neo mummy friends took me out of the hospital and down the road to a café for my birthday for lunch. Even though I felt guilty and selfish being away from my baby celebrating, *that* was a bit special to me.

For Easter, the nurses made cards from the babies and stamped each card with each individual baby's footprint for each mum; and a group called "Butts on Bikes for Prems" came through and gave every baby a hand knitted bunny. The whole ward was also transformed with colour on Easter Sunday – each baby was swaddled in either a bright coloured rabbit or chicken print blanket instead of the sea of regulated white. It was touching to think they went out of their way to make a difficult time more bearable, even if it WAS only for one day, because just that splash of colour lifted everyone's spirits.

For Mother's Day, the nurses also did the same with the cards and the Premmie Support group "Women Who Have Been There" came in and gave every mum a little goodie gift bag and a delicious cupcake.

I might just detour here and say how soul saving Jen (the founder of "Women Who Have Been There") and the other mummies are … they have all had babies go through the Neo, and they understand better than anyone what it's like – which is the whole reason they started the support group in the first place.

I met Jen a few weeks into my Neo journey at a time when I was particularly vulnerable; I had been walking around constantly in tears and a daze, trying to get a grip on everything, and to talk it out with her and get it off my chest and know she knew exactly what I was feeling really helped. Jen and the other ladies of the group make regular visits to the ward to offer support to whoever needs it, and also has a closed site on Facebook to continue the support post Neo (which has turned out to be my lifeline). Its online members are faceless avatars that are quick to offer friendship, advice and opinions. Other women WHO HAVE BEEN THERE, and personally "GET" what it is you are going through. It's a communal soft place to land and lick your wounds after such a traumatic time. It's a veritable One Stop where you can satiate your hunger for learning about all things Prem. A place to vent, share milestones, and basically seek much needed comfort from like-minded women as oneself, struggling to adjust after living life inside a Neonatal Unit.

CHAPTER SIX

As well as the day-to-day dealings with Aidan, my OWN health also took a hammering.

First, there was the blood clot in my leg. That lasted for nearly three months. I had to re-visit the doctor a couple times for the clot, and ended up being put on antibiotics because it had turned septic. At its worst, it hurt to walk because of where it was (just behind the right knee and to the left), and it constantly itched and burned like fire.

I got nipple thrush, which I put up with for three weeks before it was diagnosed as Such by a lactation consultant (I had just thought the constant pain and bleeding, peeling nipples was all part and parcel of the constant three hourly milk expressing on the machines …).

I suffered with the thrush for the better part of nine weeks before we got on top of it with antibiotics and creams. I've never known something so painful and cruel, which ALSO meant Aidan had ANOTHER thing to be treated for as well. Just ONE MORE guilt inducing factor, because YET AGAIN it was MY fault that he required additional medicines.

Then, I got mastitis. That was yet ANOTHER course of antibiotics!!! I was very miserable. I was always in tears. Nature gives you everything your body needs to conceive and sustain life, yet it seems to turn around and attack itself at will and make life very hard.

And THEN, in my own clumsiness, I was walking back to the flat one night and fell UP a flight of stairs – and bruised my ribs and one of my knees (and my ego!). My fall required a doctor's visit because I was having difficulty breathing and was in constant pain each time I took a breath. I was SO embarrassed having to explain it to the doctor. I bet they hear those sorts of things all the time … "I fell down some stairs" or "I ran into a door" . But I DID! I really did! And I felt so STUPID.

I also had visits to the doctor to have the Whooping Cough booster as is recommended for new parents and immediate family members, and the annual FluVac. By this time, I wasn't AS petrified of needles – I'd gotten used to them. I didn't LIKE having them, but kept reminding myself that it was for Aidan's benefit. And I would have walked over broken glass for him if I was told it would help him.

Up until I fell pregnant and gave birth, I couldn't even remember the last time I had even seen a doctor – it was probably for my last smear test – NOW it seemed like I was seeing one every WEEK! I felt like a car wreck and a walking pharmacy. And I was STILL having stomach pains around the navel. While in Flinders, I saw a doctor who sent me for an ultrasound but it came back with 'no known cause' for the pain I was experiencing. I'm sure they all thought it was ' just in my head '.

It wasn't until eight months later, after seeing my OWN doctor, that I found out I had an umbilical hernia. I felt like giving up. It was just one thing after another.

My emotional state was completely shot. I was alone, raw, sad, angry, resentful, grieved, depressed, confused – but most of all, I felt like a huge failure.

Life in a Neo Ward is, as I have already said, an intense emotional rollercoaster. Every positive step forward is celebrated, but every step backward (which seemed to outweigh the positives) left me absolutely shattered.

And to feel the physical nearness, but impossible distance of your baby … it's such a heart-breaking contradiction. Or the weeks where your baby doesn't improve/move forward, but doesn't lapse backward – just stays on a plateau – they were the hardest because it felt like no progress was being made at all. The nurses would joke and say, "We've never sent a baby straight from the Neo to school," but some days I started to wonder if we would EVER leave there. From the moment you step over the threshold into a Neonatal Unit, it's like you have been transported into another universe. The sights, smells and sounds are something you will never forget, even long after you have left it.

In his time in the NNU, Aidan had two blood transfusions, phototherapy for jaundice, courses of antibiotics for infections, medication to close a PDA in his heart, numerous cranial ultrasounds, ECGs, lung X-rays, and the ghastly eye tests each fortnight (to test for R.O.P) and almost daily blood tests. He went through all the levels of oxygen support (intubation, CPAP, HiFlo, LoFlo) for a total of seven weeks until he didn't need it anymore. From being fed via a drip and Perfuser machine, to a nasalgastric tube and eventually to being breastfed. Before we were discharged/transferred from Flinders, we were invited to participate in a BILI BLANKET trial, which was in direct conjunction with the phototherapy they use for jaundice, specifically, as I understood it, monitoring how much the phototherapy affected the baby's body temperature, so that they could determine whether a prem's temperature rises were related to the use of UV lamps, or from onset of infection; and being able to distinguish the two would mean a change in preventative medicine protocol (the use of antibiotics as a precautionary method) and as such, this trial could only be done on healthy prem babies, so as not to skew the results. As it was non-invasive, I was happy to let Aidan be included in the trial.

There was another trial we were asked to be involved in, A Core Temperature Trial; but it involved having a tiny probe with a thermometer attached and inserted orally down into his tummy – but I didn't allow it as I thought he already had enough gastric tubes to deal with.

In the scheme of things, and compared to some of other prems there at the time, we readily acknowledge that Aidan got off lightly with his health issues as a result of his extreme prematurity. We were very, very lucky.

When Aidan was thirteen weeks old, in our thirteenth week at Flinders (and he was BORN on the thirteenth – as was I (but a different month) – Lucky number thirteen!); we were finally transferred back home to the Mt Gambier Hospital; and my husband got to hold our son for the first time. That was such a tender moment for me – to witness that first cuddle. I knew what MY first cuddle felt like after having had to wait for five days after giving birth to hold my son. But having had to wait for thirteen WEEKS … placing our son in my husband's arms was a moment I will never forget. He just sat there for ages, staring at him in wonderment and not moving in case he hurt him. It was nothing short of magical. I cried tears of pure joy. At last my little *family* was together and complete.

After another week stay in the Mt Gambier Hospital, we finally brought our baby home for the first time. He was now the size of a small new-born, but was actually a bit over three months old. It was surreal.

Coming home was bittersweet. All I had wanted was to get out of the hospital scene and to have my baby to myself in my own home. But in reality, I was scared to death at the prospect. Hospital had become my safe place. I missed not having the 24/7 nursing care. If anything went wrong, they were there instantly and dealing with it.

And ironically, all the leads and monitors with their constant beeping that I had once despised, I now yearned for. They had visually assured me that Aidan was still breathing and that his little body was doing what it was meant to be doing. I had relied heavily on those machines.

I was still worried about Aidan's ability to breast feed, as he had only had his gastric tube removed the day before we were transferred back to the Mt Gambier Hospital. I adamantly refused to bottle feed, as we had (had) a couple dusky episodes in Flinders with bottle feeding because Aidan just couldn't get a handle on how to co-ordinate the all-important suck, swallow and breathing skill at the same time – and as a result, a couple of times he choked and stopped breathing. It was scary, especially since I was the one bottling him on one of those occasions. From then on, I saw bottles as evil, and I got cold sweats and panicky if I was coerced into giving him one. We had been having daily visits from a speech pathologist in Flinders in the last couple of weeks, to help Aidan learn to breastfeed. Our breastfeeding still wasn't fully established, and I worried about his weight gain. Weight gain in Flinders is such a big thing, and the babies are weighed every two days. Every gram gained was a triumph. While he was in Flinders, I would set my alarm and get up and call the NNU in the wee hours of a morning from the flat, just to check what that day's weight gain had been. In one day back in the Mount Gambier Hospital, his weight gain had turned to a loss.

But the locum paediatrician wasn't worried. He didn't want regular weighs.

And, all along, Aidan had (had) issues using his bowels. In Flinders, they don't Like Prem's going more than forty-eight hours without a motion. So, every two days Aidan would have a suppository to help him poo. Back in the Mount Gambier Hospital, it was going on day seven since his last movement. I was getting distraught. But I was told it was fine, that breastfed babies can go for up to two weeks without a bowel movement. They weren't concerned that this had been an issue. I was so worried something bad would happen once I got him home if it wasn't addressed and managed before we left hospital. But I felt like I was being treated like an over protective first time mum who didn't know what the hell she was on about. They even sent a doctor in to talk to me about my high levels of "anxiety". But the bottom line was, the change in professional care had me alarmed. Everything I had seen and witnessed in Flinders was dismissed and brushed under the carpet now. Had

I not had a Premmie, I would have been none the wiser. This would have all been normal and par for the course.

But the fact was – I HAD. And I was concerned for Aidan's well-being.

At home, it was quiet – too quiet. In the beginning, I kept constantly checking him every five minutes to make sure he was still alive. I would sit next to him and watch his chest rise and fall to be satisfied he was still breathing. If I couldn't see any movement, I would hold my finger under his little nose to feel for warm air being exhaled. A few times, in sheer panic, I grabbed him up to wake him. I was a nervous mess.

I had set his bassinette up in the lounge room, where the slow combustion fire was, and slept on the couch right next to him. I had multiple baby video monitors set up at various angles to keep added watch over him and took a handset with me whenever I had to leave the room. I kept the ambient temperature in the lounge at a nice twenty-seven degrees, and took Aidan's temperature every hour to start with; eventually relaxing my checks to four hourly. Surprisingly, I sorely missed the regimented, controlled atmosphere of the NNU. So much so, and to have SOME sense of control, I printed up a spreadsheet and continued to chart everything on an hourly basis like they do in Flinders – his temperature checks, feeding times, nappy changes, medications given.

I was *home*, but I felt so incredibly lonely and out of sorts. I felt like a stranger in my own house. In between feeds and nappy changes, I didn't know what to do with myself. And I missed all the Neo mums I had become firm friends with. They had travelled the same journey as I had, and we had supported each other daily while we were there. We looked out for each other, and I fondly remember one of them bringing me take-away food leftovers one night after she and her hubby had gone out for tea – she knew I would skip tea just to be with Aidan, so she delivered me food, and an iced coffee, to be satisfied that I would eat! I also had breakfast delivered one morning by the hubby of another when he went out to do a Macca's run. And if any of us had made or bought tea, and there were leftovers in the flat fridge, we would leave notes for each other to "Please help yourself." Even though we were all on the grounds at Flinders somewhere or constantly down with our babies, we were each going about our own little worlds each day because our babies would be in different bays, or upstairs in the Satellite Nursery – but we would keep in contact with each other by text messages just to make sure we were all doing okay. I really, truly missed these ladies and the moral support we had given each other. My heart ached for them. I also missed the conversations with the nurses. I had made some nice friends with a few of them who were happy to extend their friendship to me beyond Aidan's care.

I had been told by the doctors, both those in Flinders and Mount Gambier that due to his prematurity and compromised immune system, to be vigilant with Aidan's exposure to any and all illnesses – including the common cold. At least THAT was one thing they all agreed on. I was so scared of him getting sick and ending up back in hospital that I only left the house if and when I absolutely had to.

My ventures out of the house was limited to the weekly grocery shopping, and to take Aidan down to the local Child and Family Health Services office for his weekly weigh ins. I even went as far as to looking into online shopping and home delivery in my area, and to purchasing a set of baby scales, just so I wouldn't have to leave the house at all. But of course, neither was available in my area.

The grocery shopping had now become a two person job because of my paranoia *of* him catching something due to germs. I refused to use the baby holders in the trolleys; opting to leave Aidan in his capsule and put the capsule in the trolley – but not before I had wiped the trolley handle down with anti-bacterial wipes first. So I needed my husband to push the other trolley for food. I carried those anti-bacterial wipes and the Aquim gel with me wherever I went. I bought silicone "Your germs are too big for me – Please do not touch me" signs off a baby site on the internet, to hang on his capsule and pram. I knew people were thinking I was going overboard, but THEY hadn't had to see, live and feel what I had whilst in the Neo Ward for three months. People think that just because you have left hospital that your baby is "out of the woods" and that all is as it should be now – but that's not quite true. With it, comes the *fear* (of their continued health outcome), the WORRY (of quality of life regarding their development and ability to cope with certain situations), the continued 'Follow-ups' back at Flinders for many years, which leaves you feeling like you are still in limbo and STILL have no control, and the wrongly assumed stigma that your baby isn't quite 'normal'… being a Prem ISN'T a negative affliction. They are just like any other baby – they just take a longer route with more speedbumps and potholes to get where they need to go. Having felt I had already failed my baby once – I vowed to protect Aidan as best I could from here on in, and at all costs.

My days for the following months were spent, for the most part, inside my lounge room walls. Attending to, nursing and cuddling Aidan. Even when I wasn't feeding him, I kept him in my arms and just sat with him on the couch. I had a primal need to have him close at all times. I felt I had a lot of time to make up for; from when he was in Flinders for all those many weeks when he was in his humidicrib and I couldn't cuddle him like a normal mum could. I spent so much time in my lounge room that I could tell you what time of the day it was, pitifully, by what TV program was on.

I printed up a "RULES" list for visitors and stuck it to my front door: They must *have* had this year's Flu Vaccine, not recently been around sick people, not currently be sick/or recently been sick themselves, be non-smokers… And we requested that *no* children of school age visit; because even the doctors agreed that children were, inadvertently, the biggest carriers of illness and germs. We couldn't risk it. Aidan had already been through enough.

I think a lot of people took this personally, because not a lot of people visited once we were home. That hurt, but we couldn't make exceptions just because I was *feeling* down and lonely. We came to the conclusion if people couldn't respect our *requests* and the reasons for them, then we didn't want them to visit. Aidan's immune system was low and compromised due to him being born an extreme prem; so Aidan's health and well-being was our top priority.

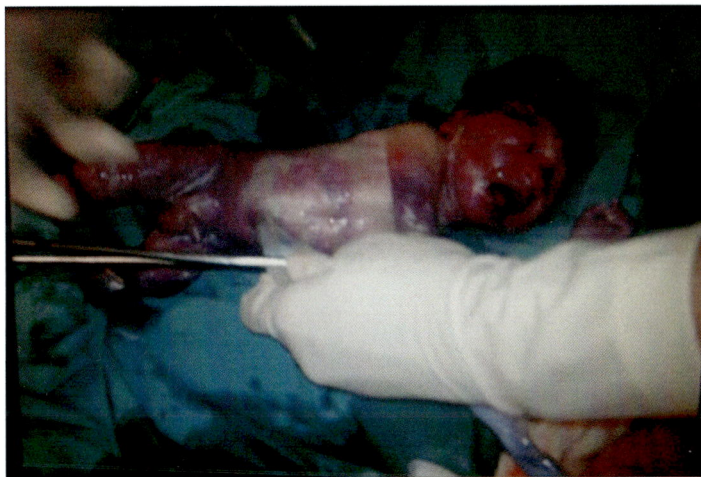
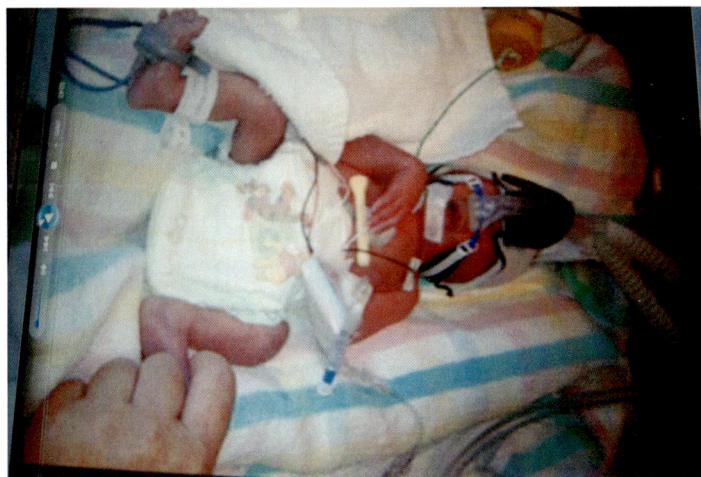

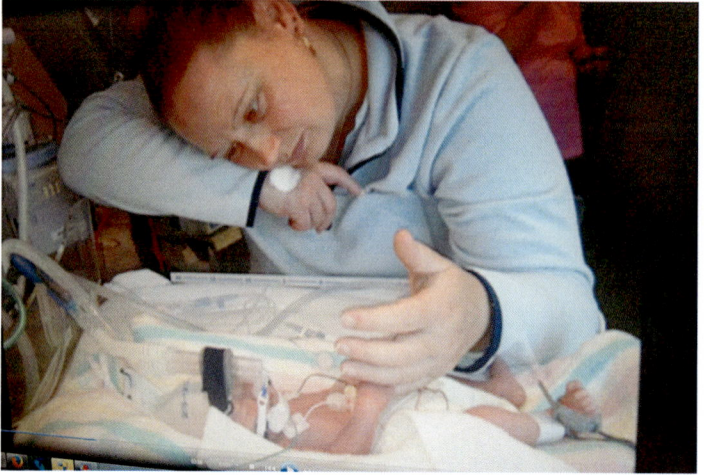

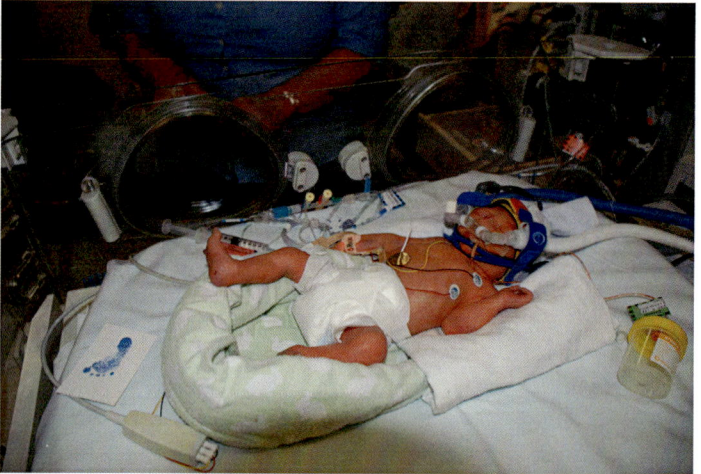

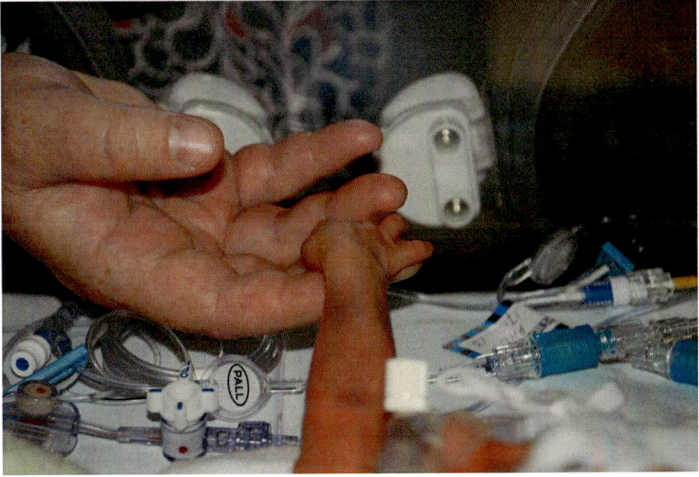
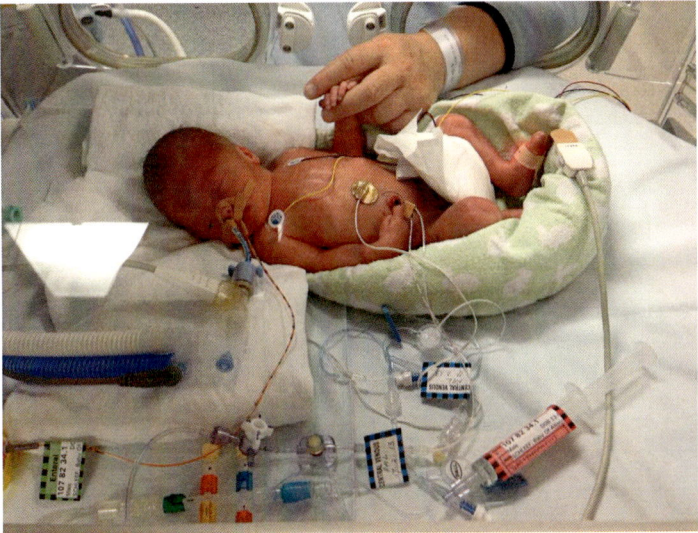

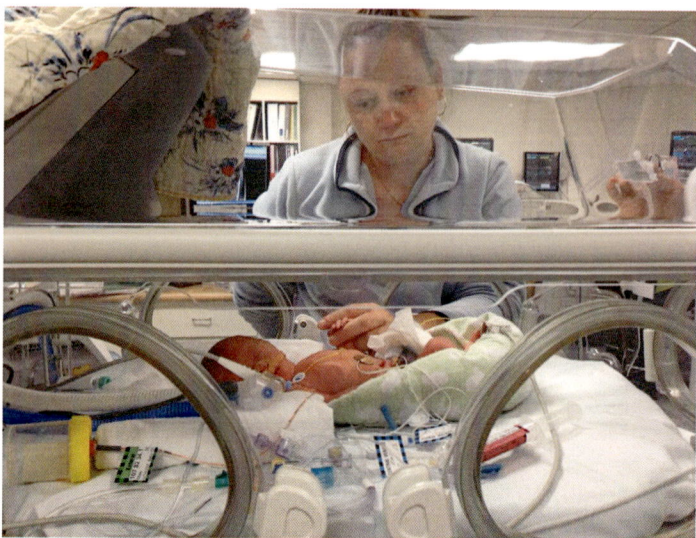
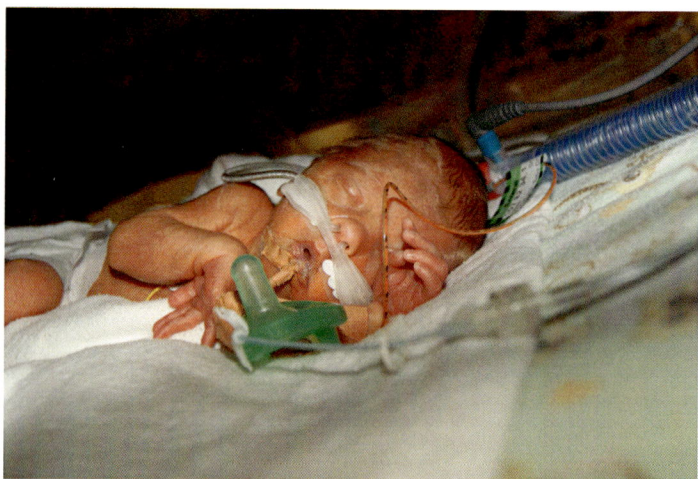

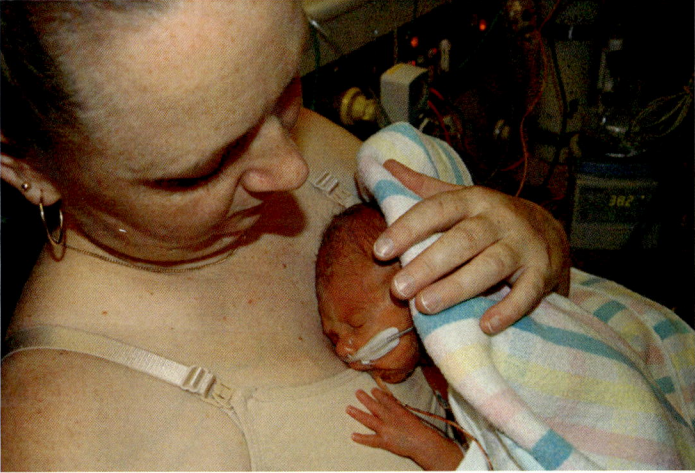

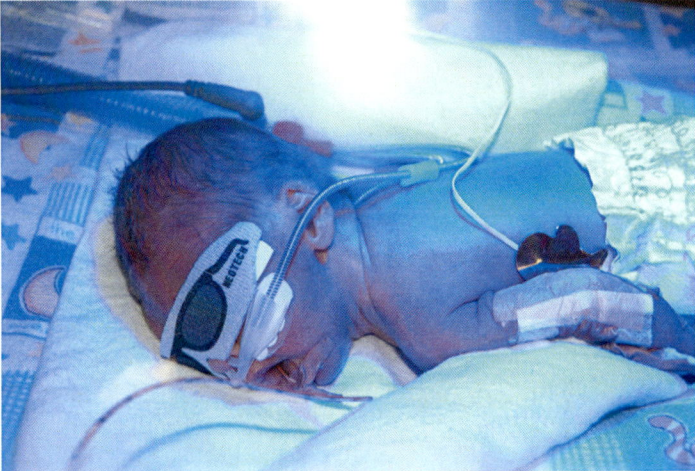

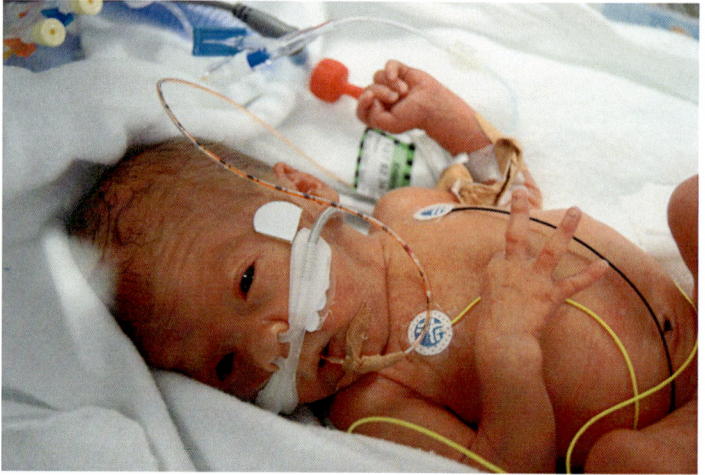

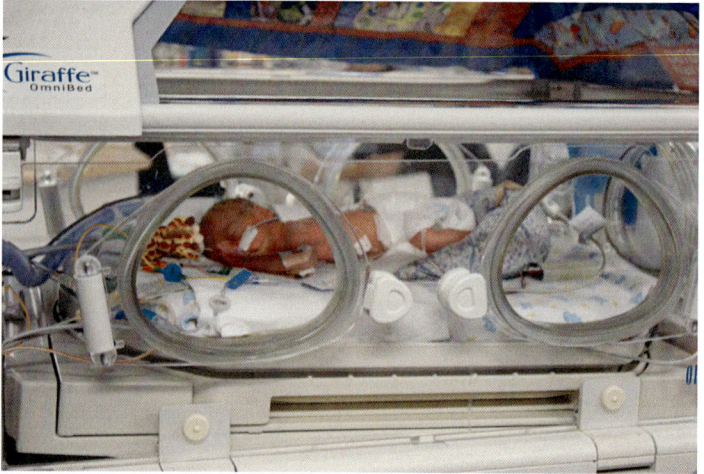

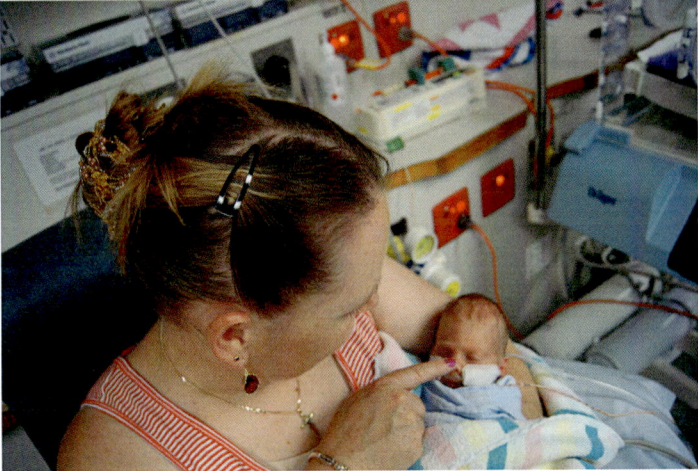
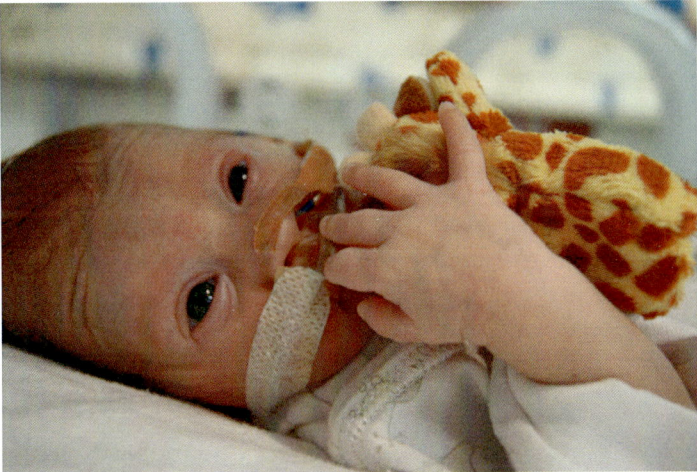

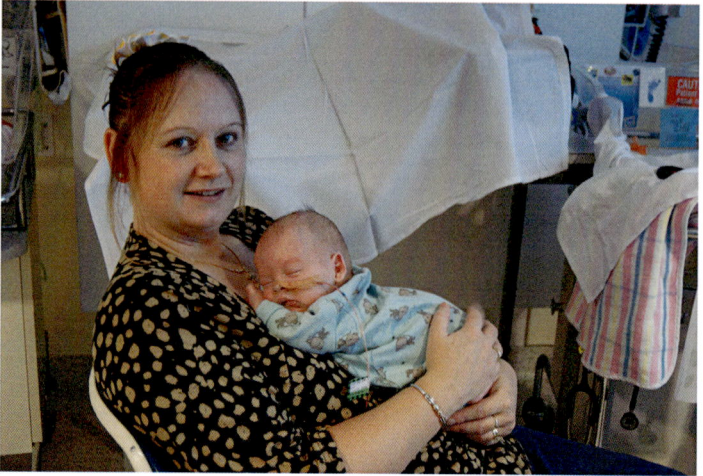
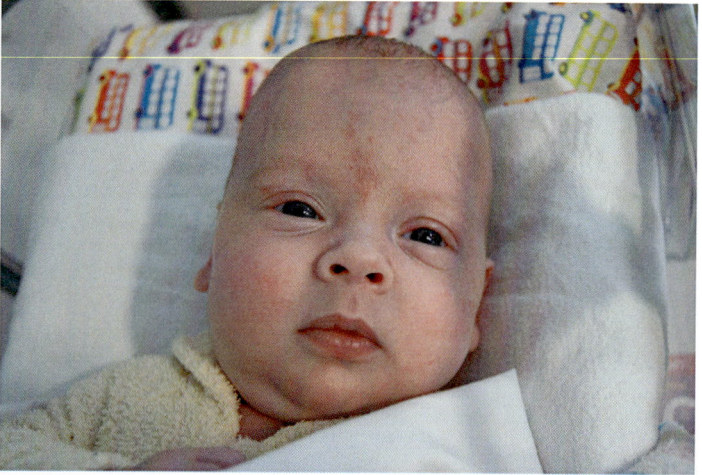

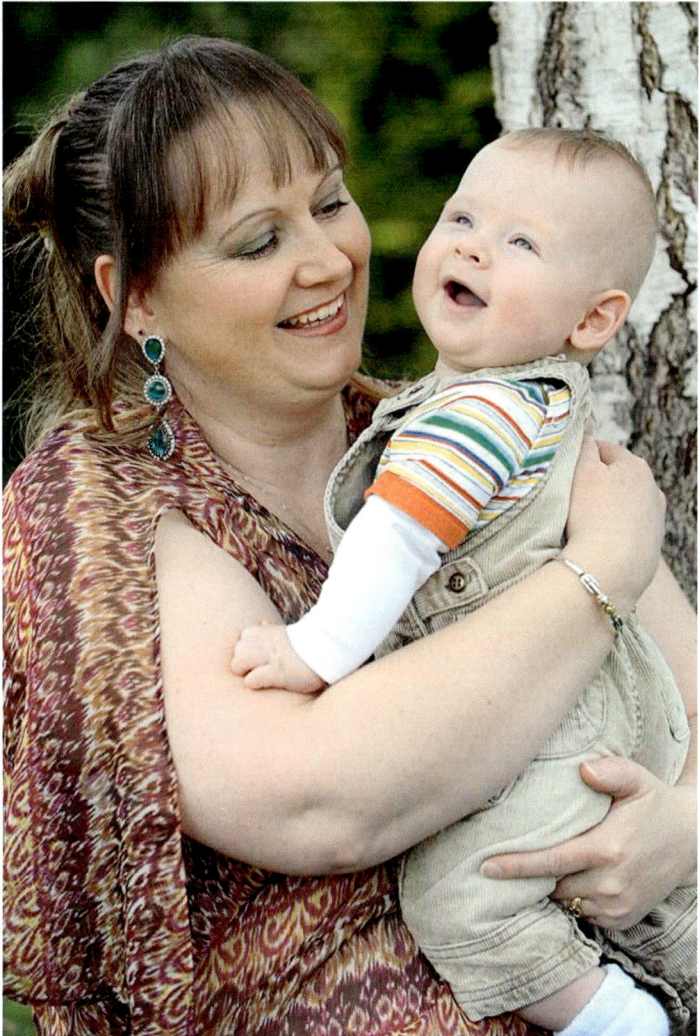

Picture Courtesy of Joanna Fincham Photography, South Australia

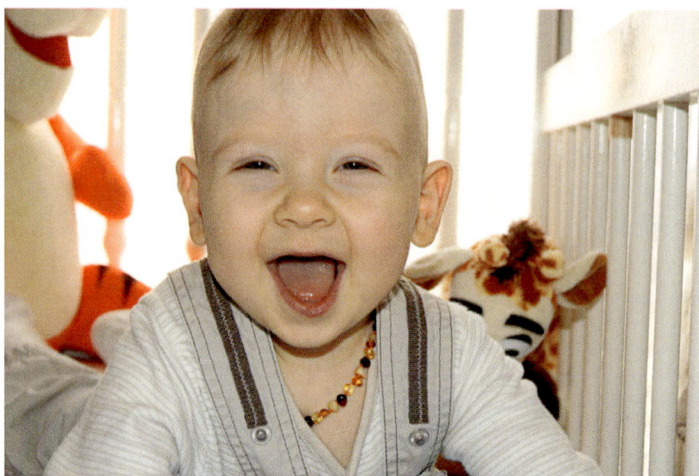
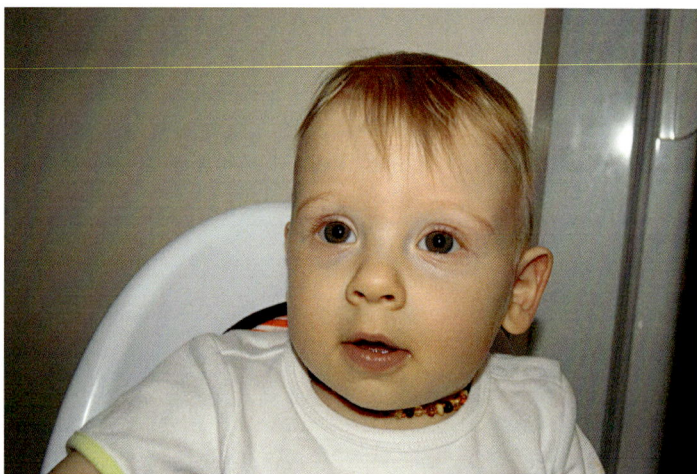

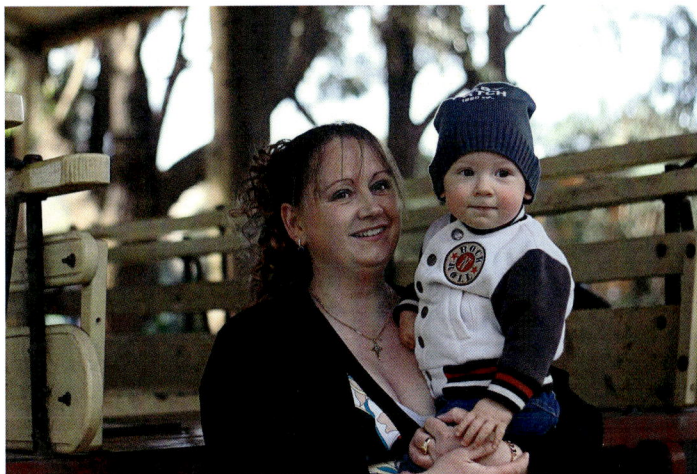
Photo by Memories by Katie

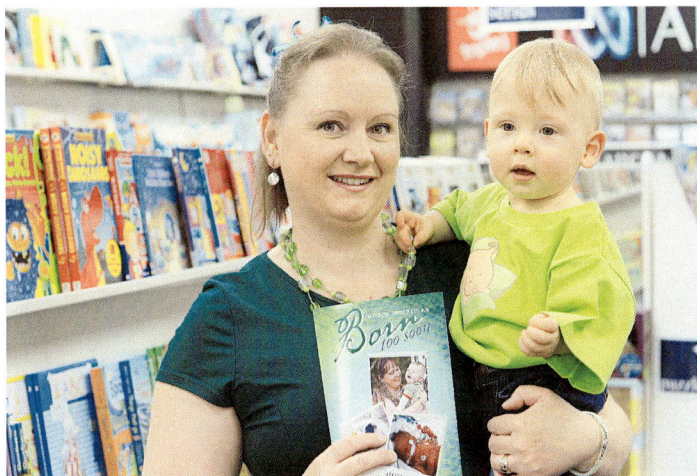
Picture Courtesy of The Border Watch, Mount Gambier, South
Australia

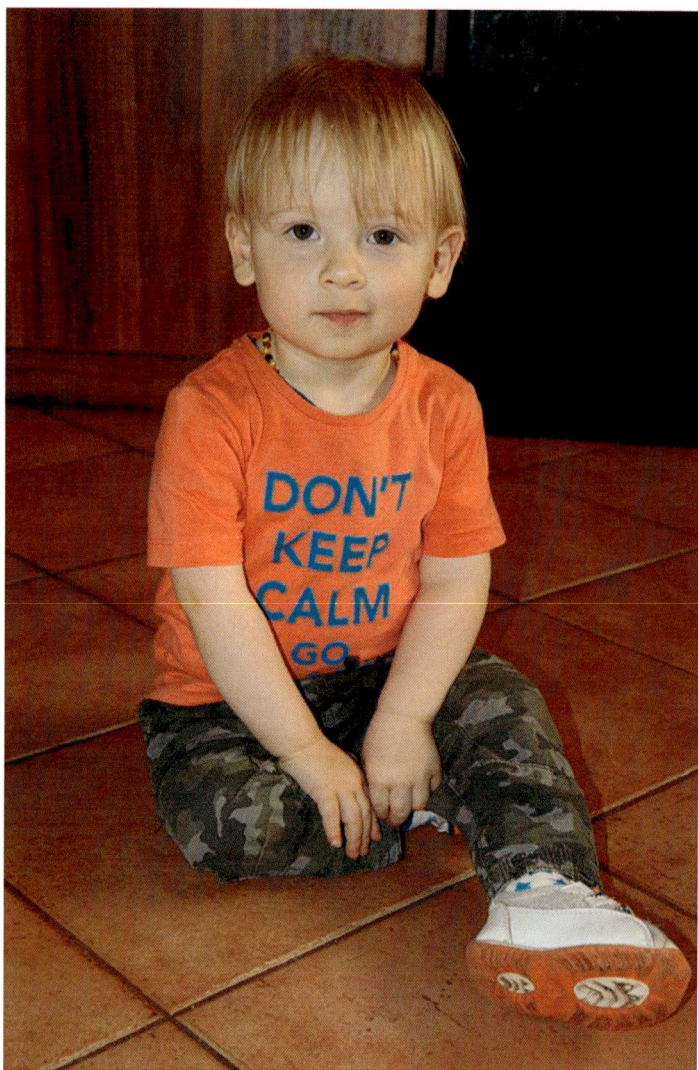

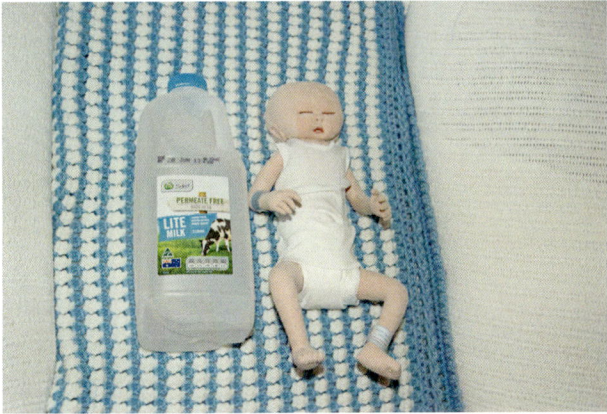

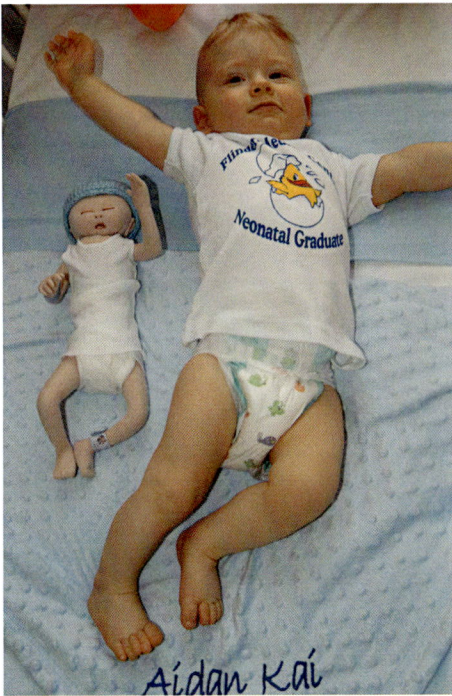

Aidan Kai

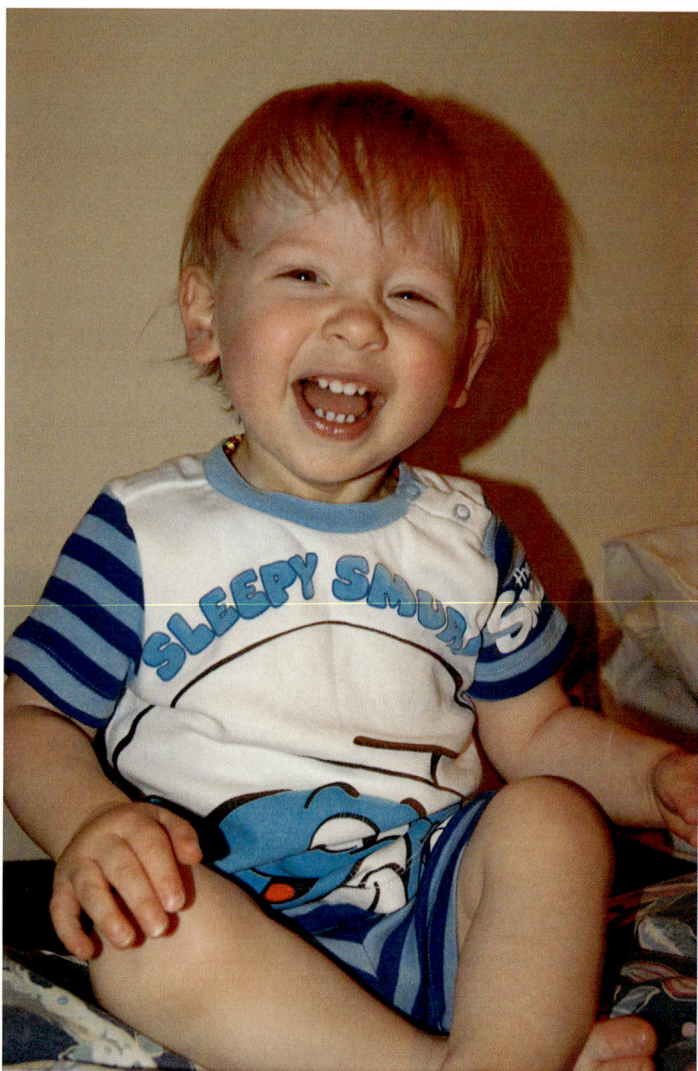

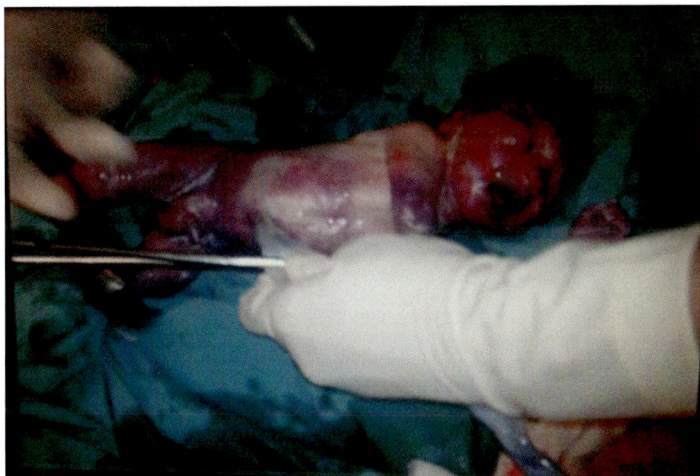
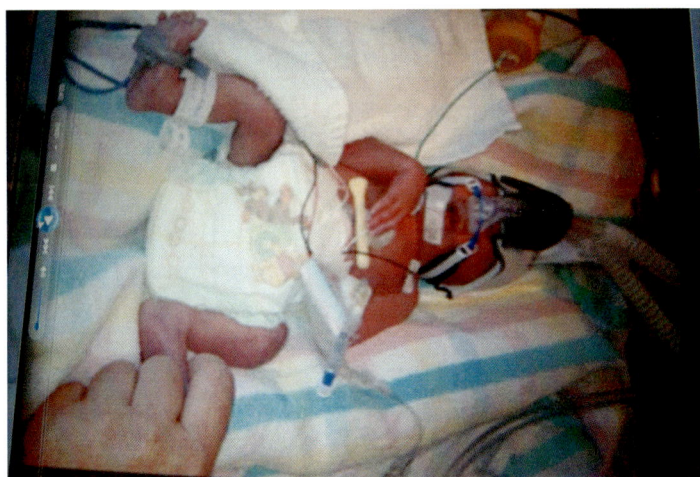

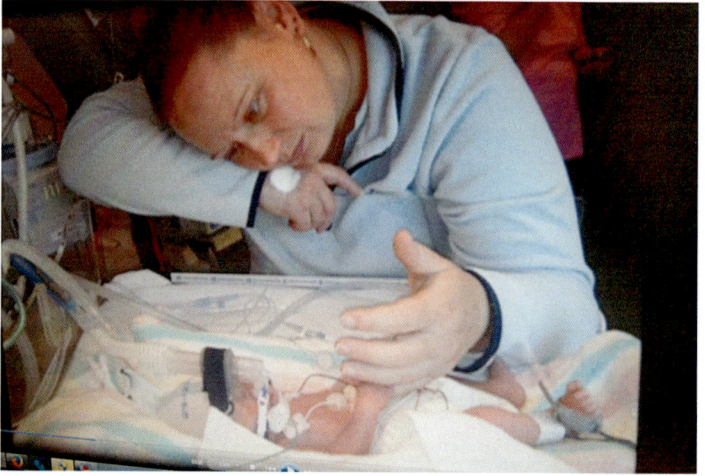

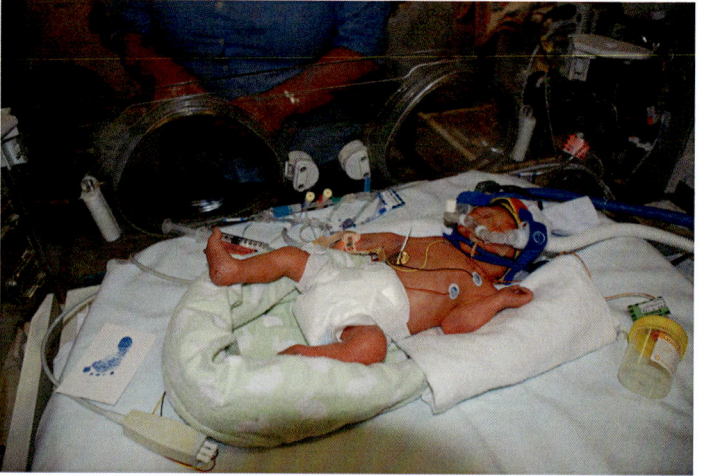

CHAPTER SEVEN

I think this is when my Postnatal Depression started to really take hold.

I had (had) so much support from my family and friends when I was up in Adelaide with Aidan in Flinders, and it seemed to fall by the way side once we were home. Whether this was my warped sense of perception or actual reality, I'm not sure, but surely, little by little, the daily text messages to see how we were, stopped. The daily phone calls stopped. The visits went from daily to weekly to monthly ... I felt like we had been abandoned. Like they thought the "crisis" was now over, now that we were out of hospital. I started to struggle big time. I was, once again, always in tears.

I had enough sense of mind to know that the world didn't revolve around Aidan and me, and that they had their OWN lives to live. I scolded myself for constantly feeling needy, and told myself I was being self-centred and selfish. Yet, irrationally, I still couldn't help but feel like I didn't matter anymore, like I wasn't a priority.

Like they didn't care. I needed someone to talk to; a shoulder to cry on. I just longed for some adult company and conversation. I was slowly languishing.

I kept re-playing in my mind, over and over, images from when Aidan was in his humidicrib. I still distinctly felt the same feelings I had felt from all the activity in the Neo. Felt the heartache of our whole journey. I could still vividly see the muted lights of the corridors and hear the hum of the vending machines as I would walk back from the Neo to the flat late at night.

Up the stairs from one floor to the next, my own footsteps echoing in the deserted hallways, pressing the after-hours button to security to be let out of the hospital.

Listening to the birdsong (wild nectar feeding lorikeets that I specifically relate to as indigenous to Adelaide), during the daylight hours, and the smell of the hot pavement and warm wind as I walked down from the flats to the hospital. Seeing the massive container ships on the ocean horizon at Glenelg to the left beyond the staff carpark on those daily treks down. Or hearing all the noises and smells from the hospital kitchen and cafeteria as I would pass it on my way back in early in the mornings; pangs of hunger ignored by my driving need to see my baby. I could still feel the emptiness and pain I had felt every time I would look out from the balcony of the flat late at night to the distant glimmer of hospital lights, knowing that (that) small expanse of asphalt and soft, almost eerie glow of orange night lights, was what was between me and my son. Or the heart palpitations I would feel every time I would hear the soft thud-thud of the Medstar Helicopter landing on the hospital roof helipad, or an ambulance siren signalling yet another emergency. It's amazing how just the memory of these things can take your breath away and make your eyes prick with tears.

The intense loneliness and despair I felt THEN, I also felt NOW. I was just so incredibly sad; all the time, for no apparent reason. And I couldn't shake the feelings of being useless; the guilt of my body failing to carry my baby to term and him having to go through what he did.

I felt like a failure. Some days – even for a week at time – I wouldn't get dressed.

I stayed inside in my PJs and dressing gown and slippers and devoted every minute to Aidan and his needs. I didn't see any point getting dressed – I didn't have any visitors, and I wasn't going anywhere.

I missed my Neo mummy friends. We were keeping in contact via Facebook, but it wasn't the same as BEING there with them. Sometimes, I wished we were still in Flinders and I was living back in the flat – just for their company. But then, thinking of being back in Flinders gave me the feeling of being suffocated. My thoughts and feelings were so contradictory, that I thought I was going mad.

I kept obsessing of all the things I'd NOT had; like the beauty of my baby bump not blossoming to full term; of not having had the 3D ultrasound package I had booked in for; of not having the pregnancy photo shoot I'd planned; of not having had a baby shower; and most importantly, for not having Aidan's birth as celebrated as it should have been. I have found that premature births are not met with the same unbridled enthusiasm as that of a Term baby, and that people are unsure whether to congratulate you or offer their commiserations. If they DO go out of their way to welcome your new addition, it is with trepidation and some degree of reserve. Perhaps this is because they just don't know what to expect or say, given the sombre nature surrounding that of a prem baby.

Even when we had been transferred back to the Mount Gambier Hospital, none of my friends or extended family bothered to come visit us. Privately, I had indulgently entertained in my mind that our arrival back to the Mt Gambier Hospital would be met with a small gathering out the front of the hospital with balloons to mark such a huge milestone – a 'Welcome Back/Welcome to the World Aidan' kind of fanfare. Instead, I feverishly drove back from Adelaide in the early hours of that morning, so I would be there when Aidan was transferred. But there were delays with his flight, so I ended up sitting at the hospital alone, frantically waiting for his return, into the early evening. There were no trumpets. There were no meet and greet. I sat there, once again, alone.

Notably the only people that did visit were my dad, my sister, my mum and Nana – and much to my surprise, a mate of my husband's that he had grown up with and we'd hardly seen since the day that we'd been married.

For all of these things, I had deep-seated misgivings and I felt sorely slighted.

And it wasn't just the whole Neo journey that made me depressed. I also had to struggle daily with the feelings I was having with not working anymore. This was the first time since I had left school to start my career, that I wasn't in the workforce, and I was having a hard time dealing with the fact that I was no longer contributing financially to the household. I felt so inadequate; like I had lost my identity somehow.

Once again, I felt like everything was out of my control. Sure, my husband and I *had* talked about, and agreed, that I would quit my job completely and stay home to raise our baby until school age, but it turned out to be easier said than done. I had always been independent, and I just couldn't get my head around the fact I was no longer employed, and I lost that feeling of being an equal in our relationship.

I felt like I was now a nobody. I lost all my self-confidence. I was struggling to keep up with the housework, and felt I was letting my husband down. I wasn't working now, so I shouldn't have any excuse NOT to keep the house tidy. But some days Aidan demanded so much of my attention, all I did was sit on the couch and feed and cuddle him. My husband said it didn't matter, but to ME it did. I used to be able to multi-task – I had run multiple commercial kitchens WITH STAFF for half my life, for crying out loud! Now, I couldn't even keep one little house. I felt like I was no longer capable of doing anything.

Even driving in my car after our hospital stay turned out to be traumatic.

On my trips home throughout our hospital stay, I would listen to my favourite PIT BULL CD and have the volume turned up loud – to keep me awake; and to feel the beat of the music to take my mind off everything. But now, hearing that same CD play; I can be driving around town and suddenly realise I am crying. I can remember with startling clarity, the emotions I had felt on those trips leaving Adelaide and then on my return trips back. Crying all the way through Adelaide and the length of the Freeway until Tailem Bend. Then driving with nothing but numbness the rest of the way home.

Hearing certain tracks, I can still envision WHERE in my drive along that long and lonely expanse of road I would have been. I think if I were to point my car in the general direction of Adelaide, and play that same CD – my car would be able to find its own way there without me behind the wheel.

And driving the car with Aidan in the backseat in his capsule left me a nervous mess, for more than a few reasons. I just lost all confidence in my ability to safely drive with him on board. I didn't like the position his head was in when he was in the capsule, and after seeing what would happen in the Neo if a baby's head flopped down chin to chest, it made me panic every time we went anywhere in the car. I would stop every few minutes and actually get out and check on him to make sure he was still breathing. It took forever to go anywhere. I found out much later, that there are little electronic devices you can get that clip onto the top of a baby's nappy that monitor their breathing and sound an alarm if they stop. One of those would have been invaluable and would have saved me so much angst!!! And I was terrified someone would cause a car crash while Aidan was a passenger.

I would sit in the driver's seat in my driveway, trying to psych myself up before I would venture out, and have mini panic attacks in the process about whether I would be able to avoid an accident if I could see one about to happen. Would I be quick enough to execute evasive manoeuvres, and keep my son safe? It wasn't just ME, anymore, I had my baby to take into account now. Those little calculated risks you take on the road – and everyone does them – such as thinking you can make the turn across the intersection before oncoming traffic reached you … I wouldn't do that anymore. I would sit stationary and wait until NO cars could be seen either side, even though it meant the drivers banking up behind me were admonishing me by way of angrily blaring their horns to vent their frustrations for me holding up traffic.

(As it was, while I was writing this book, when my son was 18mths old, an incident happened which further cemented my fears of car travel with my son on board.)

I was driving two streets away from home after heading out to run an errand one late afternoon when suddenly there was a deafening BOOM inside my car, and my son started to scream hysterically. I instinctively pulled over and was out of my seat and opening the rear door in a flash, all the while acknowledging in disbelief the fact the window beside him was now completely shattered and still making audible crackling noises like hot water being poured onto a block of ice – my only thought was to get my son out of his car seat before the window exploded in on him. I could have sworn that the perfect round hole in the window amidst the shattered glass was a bullet hole – But it turns out that I had driven past a man whipper-snippering the pedestrian strip out the front of his house and at that unfortunate exact moment, he'd flung a rock up and hit my car window. A completely innocent and an honest accident, but the trauma from it was evident for quite a few weeks after. Every time I would put my son in his car seat, he would start screaming and pointing to the window that had been shattered. Even when the window was replaced, he didn't forget. He had stopped the screaming by now, but would still point to the window and babble in low baby speak. The repair man said it was lucky the window wasn't wound down at the time – or the rock would have hit my son.

(Definitely not something I had even considered!)

Right from the start, I quite literally was scared of going anywhere in the car, that I tried NOT to, unless my husband came too – so he could drive and I could sit in the back right next to Aidan to keep an eye on him. I was still a back seat passenger when my son was twenty-two months old (habits are hard to break). And if I DID drive, I was always cautious to the extreme, and never ventured anywhere without my rearview 'babyview' mirror

Six months later, at a scheduled CAFHS appointment; a nurse gave me the EPDS Questionnaire again, and I scored 21. (I had filled one out before I gave birth and scored 8, and another just after we had initially come home from hospital, in which I scored 12. I remember that CAFHS nurse voicing her concern, but I brushed it off.) She wrote me a letter to give my doctor, to discuss with her a Mental Health Plan.* She also assured me, that no-one would take my baby just because I was depressed!!!

I had been REALLY scared about that. I would not have coped had they cited me as unfit to be a mother. I loved (and love) Aidan with all of my being.

So hearing that gave me the strength to then ask for the help I knew I needed. I HAD to do SOMETHING – in my misery I had been comfort eating and had put on 15kg *since* giving birth and coming home from the hospital scene. I now weighed more AFTER the birth of my baby than when I was pregnant.

And being stressed and depressed had made my milk supply wane considerably; forcing me to resort to formula supplement feeds. That in itself made me even more depressed. Not that I am against formula feeding, or judgemental of mums who choose not to breastfeed. We all do what we have to, as individuals and do what works for us. But after persevering through the nipple thrush and mastitis and finally establishing our breastfeeding, I felt it was the ONE thing I could actually do right. Now, after everything, I felt like my body was failing me – YET again. It had become a catch-22. Lucky for me, by then, Aidan HAD learnt to bottle feed. Or he would have gone hungry.

But after a couple visits with my doctor, and discussing my options, I decided in the interim, that I didn't want medication to help me cope better. Mainly, because I didn't want to be taking anything that would go through (what was left of) my milk supply and into Aidan.

I wouldn't even take something as benign as a Panadol unless I absolutely HAD to.

No, this was something I had to do on my own. I needed to do it myself. So long as I had the support of a few good friends and a good doctor and counsellor, I was determined I was going to lift myself out of my funk. Talking it out turned out to be therapeutic. I had a few lengthy chats with a good friend of mine, Jo, who has also suffered with depression herself, and so knew what I was feeling. Spending time with Jo left me feeling like my batteries had been replaced.

I rekindled an old friendship with a former ex-family member with whom I had once been close with, and she surprisingly turned out to be very supportive.

I went out and bought a baby-carrier and, as the days got better and the sun shone a bit more, I would baby-wear Aidan out to the local shopping centres to just window shop, and to generally get out of the confines of the house. I found that once I was out and about in a social environment, I felt energised. Sunlight and fresh air was not something I had thought much about, but it turned out I had missed it. Once I was away from home, I would not want to come back!!

I made up a Journey Photo Book. As it turned out, I still had a lot of "firsts" as visual keepsakes, after all. And these are all the more special and cherished because of the remarkable fighting spirit and resilience of Aidan behind them.

I also leaned heavily on the other premmie mum's on the closed Facebook pages.

On the night's that I couldn't sleep – which seemed to be nearly every night – I would log endless hours on the premmie support Facebook sites, reading about other people's troubles and woes to try and allay my own concerns. It always helped me because no matter how BAD I thought OUR situation had been – I would always find someone ELSE who's had been even WORSE. Not that these things are a competition – what an odious and repugnant thought – but THAT realisation helped put things into perspective. I am not the only one. It is not only about US. And as grave as things had seemed at the time – there was always someone worse off. That mantra helped keep me grounded.

I still fill out his daily charts, although I must admit, more increasingly of late I am a bit lax and end up missing a few entries. Perhaps that's a sign I am nearly ready to let that obsession go. On some days I have realised I haven't taken his temperature all day – I panic a bit and chide myself, but then realise it hasn't adversely affected him.

But what turned out to be the biggest help to me was writing my first book.

I initially wrote it in the hopes it would give other mums comfort and encouragement, and strength to face each day. But after reading it myself, it made one thing abundantly clear – Despite all the hurt and heartache and waylaid plans, I AM truly blessed.

Yes, my baby had a scary and rocky start to life and things didn't go according to Allison's Law (as is my need to be an unwitting control freak).

But at the end of the day, I have a healthy, thriving little boy; and I am acutely aware that some Neo mum's don't walk away that lucky.

So I have come to think maybe I DON'T have the right to feel slighted, ripped off or sad and sorry for myself after all. We have MORE than enough reason to celebrate.

And I am reminded of this, every time I look at our beautiful son. He is my inspiration. His existence gives validation to my life and has taught me the true meaning of *love*. Right from the moment I saw those two pink lines on the test strip – I loved him. My sister used to tell me of the saying – 'A woman becomes a mum as soon as she falls pregnant; but a man only becomes a dad the day the baby is born.' I guess that is relatively true. Women bond with their baby as soon as they know there is a *life* growing inside them. Men can't bond with the baby until it physically exists. And to then be deprived of proper contact with your baby only further deepens and strengthens that bond, sometimes to the point of obsession. At least, this was true for me.

The nurses tell you that one way to look at your premmie situation is that it is a privilege to watch and witness your baby grow; day by day, week by week, in front of your very eyes, instead of hidden away inside you.

If you can put everything else aside, look past the tubes and nasal prongs and machines, past the profound effects of your emotional rollercoaster; Then on reflection I would have to wholeheartedly agree – there is no denying the sheer fascination, awe and beauty of watching an unfinished foetus morph into a beautiful baby.

We truly are, fearfully and wonderfully *created*.

CHAPTER EIGHT

13.2.13 (Day 1)

Late PM – Came down from 4SMG ward with nurse to be reunited with you. Got the shock of my life to see you in the Neonatal Ward. Didn't even know such a ward existed, or on such a large scale – so, so many babies; so many life bubbles. So upsetting to see you hooked up to all those machines and have so many tubes and wires coming out of you. It's just not natural. I feel like my heart has been ripped out.

I am crying openly, and I don't care who sees me. I have not even had you in my arms yet. I am still not allowed to hold you. The most I can do is touch your hand through the portholes of your humidicrib, and only after sanitising my hands. Hand sanitiser pumps are everywhere, on every bench, on every wall. It scares me beyond belief to see you this way. To not be able to do anything except sit beside you and watch your tiny chest rise and fall as you breathe. You don't move much, just lay there silent. They tell me it's from the morphine you had for the plane trip over, to stabilise you. My eyes prick with tears in fear when your machines start to alarm. My God – what is happening to you?? The nurse is attending to you, checking this, checking that. A part of me wants to run; I can't bear to see you like this. But I can't move. I can't bring myself to leave.

You need me, even if it's to just watch over you. I am told I have 24/7 access to the ward, so I will sit here for as long as I can until I truly can't bear it anymore. I must be strong, for your sake. You are all that matters. There are two babies to one nurse in NICU.

15.2.13 (Day 3)

Heard you cry for the first time since being here this morning. It was so quiet and muffled by your bubble that at first I didn't realise it was you. Your nurse asked me for my permission to give you a dummy to help your suck reflex. It's a green one, and it covers half your face. Got to *talk* with Dr. R. today when he did the rounds. Aside from the usual host of health issues most premature babies have, among them is Chronic Lung Disease and an open PDA (heart valve).

And whilst you may LOOK like your daddy, but you have MY blood type! Looks will change, but your blood type won't!!

You always seem to have the hiccups, and in such a small body, it looks painful to watch.

Your nurse explained to me that hiccups in Prems is an indication that you are not coping *with* life outside the womb; or too much handling and stimulation. Whenever you get too overwhelmed, your little body is wracked with hiccups. Oh my Little Man XXX

17.2.13 (Day 5)

8.00pm – Just got back from Mt Gambier from collecting my car and bringing your pa back to stay with me in the flat. Haven't even unpacked the car yet – I couldn't wait a minute longer to see you!!! Got the BEST news when I came into the NNU – I can FINALLY have my first cuddle!!!!! Your central lines in your belly button were removed today, so it is now safe to hold you.

I couldn't stop crying when the nurse placed you on my chest – you are so tiny, but so perfect and so MINE! Best experience ever!! I didn't want to give you back. But your machines started to go off, and the nurse said you were getting over-stimulated and needed to go back to your pod. I feel like I have been on the happy gas! The wait to hold you was SO worth it, Lil Man. XX

19/2/13 (Day 7)

Nurse pointed out that you are officially seven days old today! One whole *week*!!

Got to change my first nappy today. Was a challenge, trying to do it through the portholes on your humidicrib. And Hellooooo sprinkler! Mummy wasn't quick enough, and the nurse had to change your whole bedding. I had to hold you up so she could do it, and I was so scared I would drop you or hurt you. I was shaking the whole time. I had my hands spread out and palms held together at the sides, and your little body fit inside. Your head was on one palm, and your little bum on the other palm. Was intrigued to see, the nappies are weighed before use, and then again AFTER use – to determine fluid output.

Ingenious. A volunteer lady sits in the Parent Room and weighs each nappy individually and writes the weight on the front of the nappy in black text.

I had a nice chat to one this morning while I had a coffee.

The volunteers do SO MUCH for the Neo Ward. They even made you a special Name card for the front of your crib. Beautiful.

Your blood tests today show you have high bilirubin (toxic waste) in your little body that you can't get rid of by yourself; so you have to do a little sunbaking under the UV lights to help break it down. They put a purple light directly over the top of your humidicrib, and you have these little Velcro sunnies on to protect your eyes. Your daddy would be chuffed! Daddy has a sunglasses fetish. Must save this "pair" of your first sunnies!!

You came off the CPAP oxygen today, and are now on HiFlo. Which means you now don't have that hat thing on with oxygen tubes that hides half your little face – it's now nasal prongs.

Also got to feed you for the first time tonight through your gastric tube! The nurses make it look so easy, but I was so nervous! Was told we always have to *check* the ID code on the side of the syringe that contains my expressed breast milk with the ID number on your gavage line – to make sure they match the right mother's liquid gold to the right baby! You are 107 82 34. 1

This is also done for every procedure performed, and every medication given.

Two nurses must check everything done to every baby, each and every time. And then it is all documented and signed.

They are increasing my milk feeds soon from 1ml every four hours to 1ml every two hours.

You also get PNS (Parenteral Nutrition Solution) and lipids (fats) through the drip in your arm. The more EBM you get the less PNS and Lipids – until eventually you will be on ALL mummy's milk only.

It still amazes me the way the nurses take out (aspirate) all the excess air from your belly on a regular basis. The hi-flo blows your belly up like a balloon, so they have to suck it back out. I watched a nurse remove ten syringes full of air one night!!! I'm always worried now that your belly will explode if they don't do this early enough or regularly!!

23/2/13 (Day 11)

6.00am – lovely Mummy cuddles. You gazed into my eyes for ages. Not that you can actually SEE yet; but it looked and FELT like you only had eyes for me. I am still nervous holding you – you are so tiny and fragile and I'm scared if I move you will slip out of the blanket and fall onto the floor. Changed four nappies today – all with added "extras." Put the first nappy on too loose. You wet the bed (my fault), and your nurse had to give you a new sheet and nest. I felt really bad, but was told it happens often. The second nappy, after fighting with your leads and cords; turned out to be back to front, so I had to start all over again!! Come on! For the love of God – it's a bloody NAPPY! How hard can it be?! (after lunch) Devastated. Came back from the flat to be told you have elevated white blood cells in your blood work today, which means the onset of infection.

So you are being put on antibiotics. You have also been having a lot of Brady's today. So your Hi-Flo has been put back up to 6ltrs. Also found out, you get a daily dose of caffeine – to help your brain stem tell your body to keep breathing.

I found that slightly amusing. Mummy loves her coffee, too.

Sitting here beside you, I gaze around the ward at all the other babies in their bubbles.

Just like you; so vulnerable, so innocent. None of you asked to be here, yet here you all are. None of this is your fault. I am so sorry my Lil' Man.

Seeing so many tiny babies on life support is so, so sad. I have to keep taking breaths.

I feel panicky. This is all so unnatural. Mummies (and some Daddies) visiting, then having to leave their babies here and go home empty handed. Heart-breaking. I cry every night I leave you.

But I am proud to say, Mummy can now sit and watch your daily heel pricks for blood tests – I even hold the cotton ball on your heel afterwards to stop the bleeding. I used to run off in horror and hide in the Parent Room while it was being done. I still don't like hearing you cry in pain. They give you sucrose before they do any procedure, to help with the pain. But it must still hurt. I hold onto your little hand and stroke your little head and talk to you until it's over.

Am told it's now MY job to do your "cares." That's where I clean your eyes and mouth, change your nappy. Saline on a cotton ball for your eyes. Sterilised Water on a Q – tip for your mouth. They don't like to disturb you too often, because SLEEP = GROWTH; so they like to do "cluster cares" every four hours – Eye Toilet, Mouth Toilet, nappy, temp check, meds. Feeds are given at the times they are due, because being fed by gastric tube requires no effort on your part and is done while you still sleep. But quickly becoming my pet hate is seeing you with the saliva bubble build up on your lips from the Hi-Flo. I clean it off every time it gets too bad – four hours or not.

How are you expected to breathe when your mouth is clogged up with foam?

You are going up to 2ml EBM every hour later today.

25/2/13 (Day 13)

6.00am – Nurse Mel told me you have put on a whopping 160gm since your last weigh in!! Weighs are every two days. She checked it twice, just to make sure.

WOW!! You now weigh 1380gm. (You lost a bit in the first week from what you weighed at birth.)

They tried to go up to 3ml EBM every hour overnight, but your little belly couldn't handle it. Your aspirates have been tinged with green; your immature belly just can't digest that volume. So back to 2ml per hour for now.

Third cranial (brain) scan is clear (of bleeds). Very relieved. Doc told me that even though they will still keep giving you regular brain scans for a few weeks, if you haven't had a bleed on the brain in the first week then it is unlikely that you will – but they keep checking just to make sure.

Your PDA (valve in heart) is still open; so they giving you medication to try and close it. If that fails, it may have to be done surgically. No no no no!

1/3/13 (Day 17)

Mummy went home for a day to see your daddy, and it broke my heart again to have to leave you. I was crying so much before I left that your nurse was concerned.

But she promised they would take good care of you.

Came back to find that you have gone from 2ml per hour up to a HUGE 7ml per hour – and going up to 8ml very soon!!! Only one more ml, and then you will be taken off the PNS and be on ALL Mummy's milk!!! Way to go, Lil' Man!!!

4/3/13 (Day 20)

You have been up and down on my milk the last few days, your little belly can't handle the volume yet. Back down to 6ml per hour. HiFlo been turned down to 2ltrs – with talk of changing to LoFlo soon. A step in the right direction. You are a bit mischievous...you keep pulling your nasal prongs out! And it's like you KNOW you're not meant to, because you grab them with your little fingers, stare at me and then pull down on them and pull them out of your nose!! And I swear you smile while you are doing it! I poke them back in, but you just keep doing it like it's a game.

(pm) – HiFlo has been removed!!! YAY! Now we can see your gorgeous little face properly. And no LoFlo – straight off the oxygen altogether! Of course, it depends on how you do without it but Ward Doc says you are doing Super Well!!!

7/3/13 (Day 23)

Your mummy had the fright of her life this morning when the doctor himself rang me.

Damn nearly wet myself when I heard his voice. But he was just ringing to tell me that you are being put back onto the HiFlo because your little body is getting tired having to cope on its own. Your nurse noticed that your skin was getting "mottled?" A sign apparently that there isn't enough oxygen circulating your body. I had a feeling it was too soon to take you off it, but far be it for ME to question their decisions. They are the experts. That's why you are here in their care.

8/3/13 (Day 24)

Had beautiful delicious early morning "fill Mummy's reserves" cuddles − for two whole hours. I never knew I could love something so much as I do you. You may still look like a prem, with a funny shaped head and spindly arms (and I can say that because I am your mummy xxxx) – but to ME, you are perfection. XXX

Came back from having a nap to find you have gone from HiFlo to LoFlo. YAY!! That's smaller nasal prongs and less air pressure coming out of them. But my milk is now being put through the Perfuser again because your aspirates have been high. Every time you seem to have some progress, you also seem to have a setback. It's very upsetting. But Ward Doc tells me that you are now essentially deemed SPECIAL CARE as opposed to Intensive Care; you are still only in NICU due to bedding and staffing issues.

9/3/13 (Day 25)

Ward Doc told me when I came in this morning that you are being moved to the Special Care (NSCU) area later today! WOW!!! That means you can also have CLOTHES on for the first time, too. There is one nurse to three babies in NSCU (that's six babies and two nurses in each bay)

13/3/13 (Day 29)

You have been in the Special Care Ward for four days now. I am a bit worried you are *getting* sick. You sound very snuffly and snotty, and you really seem to be struggling to breathe – more like gasping. I hate watching you like this. It hurts my heart. You are still on the LoFlo and still being fed via the Perfuser. EBM has now gone up to 10ml per hour. You have been having a few Desats lately, to the point where you need oxygen added to your LoFlo – but no more than 25-30% because too much oxygen can apparently damage your eyes. We had our first NIPPLE SUCK today! Consultant Doc on rounds this morning requested it, even though the nurses were of the opinion you are too young (gestational wise) to want to or be able to yet. But you proved them wrong! You latched straight on and had a few good strong sucks – Mummy is SO PLEASED, Lil' Man! What a trooper!!

15/3/13 (Day 31)

After voicing my concerns for three days now, Doc R. has ordered for you to have an NPA (boogie test) to test for Rhinovirus. I hope you are not sick. We seem to be on a plateau at the moment. One day you are doing really well, the next day you Desat constantly and need oxygen. Weight gain has slowed right down – 10gms in two days is not enough says Doc R. It should be a MINIMUM of 40gms (20gm each day). So he has ordered for CALORIES to be added to my milk, and for you to go back onto drop feeds each hour and get off the

Perfuser machine. They are hoping though that this won't overload and upset your little belly. The good news today is, you are NOT sick. So relieved!! The results of your boogie test came back negative. So they *are* telling me your sniffles is from the LoFlo, because the air in LoFlo is dry, whereas the air was moist in the HiFlo.

16/3/13 (Day 32)

Big *day* for you, Lil' Man!! Your daddy flew over just to see you! He thought you were just so precious, and he said he couldn't believe we had made you XXXXX

You were sleeping, and Daddy didn't want to disturb you by asking the nurse to get *you* out for a cuddle (but I personally think he was just too scared to hold you because you are so tiny); so we just sat beside you, watching you while I quietly explained procedures and Neo protocols to your daddy. And he watched, fascinated, as I fed you, your next scheduled milk feed through your tube. It made my eyes prick with tears, watching your daddy see you in your surroundings for the first time and seeing his awe and wonderment – and frustration. Every time your alarms went off, Daddy was like "What's happening? What's wrong? Is Aidan ok?" I was like that initially, too. But sitting with you each day has made me used to it.

I love your *daddy*. And I love *you* XX

17/3/13 (Day 33)

You started what they call "Grading Feeds" today, but they had to go back to the hourly drop feeds because your little belly couldn't handle it. 70gm weight gain since last weigh, SO MUCH BETTER than the previous 10gm!

19/3/13 (Day 35)

Another 80gm weight gain! Choofing along now!! They decided this morning on rounds to try the Grading Feeds again. You are currently on hourly feeds. The idea is to get you onto two hourly feeds, then three hourly, then four. It is a bit complicated.

It goes something like this: Currently you are on 10ml per hour. So Grading goes –

First hour, 10ml; second hour, 9ml; third hour, 11ml. Then 8ml, 12ml, 7ml, 13ml, 6ml, 14ml, 5ml, 15ml, 4ml, 16ml, 3ml, 17ml, 2ml, 18ml, 1ml, 19ml – hold for one hour, then 20ml.

Then every two hours you get a 20ml feed, and another 2ml is added each day – providing, of course, your belly can digest the volume.

So to re-cap: As of today, you are on 22mls my milk every two hours which is fortified with 85% calories and 4% polyjoules, plus you have just been put on daily Pentavite and Vitamin E (the Vit. E is an antioxidant to stop your prem body from breaking down your own red blood cells). And you are still on your daily dose of caffeine.

The nurses keep telling me how big you are getting now, but I can't see it because I sit with you and see you every day. To ME, you are still teeny tiny, only now you have chubby cheeks. Today you are 1870gm, 43cm long and your head is now 28cm in circumference. You were born 1350gm, 40cm long, 25cm head.

21/3/13 (Day 37)

We had another go at the boob this morning! What a Lil' Champion you are!! You might be little, but you know EXACTLY what to do! Nurse Chris said you seem more advanced than your 33 weeks age gestation. You have put on another 50gm. You now weigh 1920gm. Not too far off the 2kg milestone! That open crib is only a touch away!!

23/3/13 (Day 39)

WHOA!!!!!!! Came in at 6am to find you IN AN OPEN COT!!! Your overnight weigh in tipped you over the 2kg mark – you put on a whopping 130gm. FINALLY, I don't have to ASK permission to hold you now; I am allowed to pick you up when I want to (but still in keeping with their SLEEP = GROWTH policy).

Of course, you still have all your pesky cords, but they wrap you in such a way that all the cords are down the bottom of your swaddle, so it's easier to handle you. This is *such* an achievement! I have been WAITING for this day!! Now I just have to get over my fear of you sliding out the bottom of your swaddle when I pick you up! Funny, the little weird things that go through your mummy's mind!!

Going home again today to see your daddy – I have been doing this once a week for the past five weeks and I thought it would get easier each time, but it actually gets harder. I don't sleep the night before, and I am in tears all morning before I go. I cry all the way to Tailem Bend. And then am just numb and drive without really seeing. Not being able to see you or touch you or cuddle you for forty-eight hours hurts like you wouldn't believe. I call the Parent line every couple hours and talk to your nurse to check on you while I am gone; but it's not the same as BEING THERE with you. I love your daddy; and for my OWN sanity I NEED to go home to see him – but it's such a relief to get back to you. Until I physically feast my eyes on you again, it feels like I am holding my breath.

I love your daddy, but YOU are literally a part of me, and my love for you is different – its raw, its humbling, its fierce, it's pure, it's all consuming and it's unconditional.

You will probably never understand how much I love you,
Aidan Kai XXXXXXX

27/3/13 (Day 43)

Oh no – today is the day for your first Eye Test. And it's freaking me out that they *would* put such an innocent baby through such a traumatic experience. I witnessed the baby next to you have it done last week – I didn't know what was going on at first, because I keep to myself when sitting next to you (as is Neo policy) – but it was impossible NOT to hear her bloodcurdling screams. I sat beside you, with tears in my eyes, holding my breath until it was over. It was horrible to hear that tiny baby scream like that. I know it has to be done; it's a necessary evil. But you will have to forgive me, Lil' Man – *this* is one test Mummy can't stand to watch, so I can't bring myself to stay with you while it's done. I am going to wait in the Parent Room, and your nurse can come get me when it's over. Then I will cuddle you all better.

Phew – your eye test result is a good one; so far, your blood vessels are growing as they should be with no interruption. But you need these ghastly eye tests fortnightly now until the blood vessels have reached the outer rim of your eye. You poor baby.

Doc on rounds today made the decision to stop your daily dose of caffeine. I hope it's *not* too soon. Like the oxygen. And speaking of oxygen – LoFlo has been removed!! Again!! Let's see how long you last without it THIS time. They have tried to remove it a couple times already but ended up hooking you back up to it because you started to struggle and weren't ready yet. So fingers crossed!!!

28/3/13 (Day 44)

You've been off your caffeine now for a bit over twenty-four hours and so far so good. And at my request they have stopped your Gaviscon with every feed – it was binding you up something terrible. You were screaming and back arching and pushing for a poo so hard your face was going red and I thought you were going to blow your brain out.

But maybe that wasn't my brightest idea – this afternoon you started *bradying* and *desatting* again. Nurses are pretty sure it's reflux related, because it's worse just after a feed. Feeding you is not fun anymore. I get tense now every time I pour your milk down your gavage tube; because not long after, you start desatting or spewing everywhere. It never used to be like this.

31/3/13 (Day 47)

Today was meant to be my last day of work before my maternity leave started, Lil' Man.

Easter Sunday! But you had other ideas! And it's been a day of tears. Started with me waking up to find my boobs were rock hard and painful but I couldn't get any milk out when I tried to "express." And when I came down to you, you did nothing but desat after desat after desat. In the end I was so upset I went back to the flat and cried myself to sleep – it all just became too distressing to watch. When I came back down, I was told they did an FBE (full blood evaluation) on you and found out that your haemoglobin levels are really low – 76 – when they should be 130–180.

So you may be looking at having a blood transfusion. That's why you are desatting all the time. But Doc B. wants to sit it out for a bit and see if your little body will start to make its own red blood cells before they intervene. I am sorry, my Little Man. I shouldn't have been so sooky and thinking of myself and left you on your own today. I should have been here for you. I hope you can forgive me.

1/4/13 (Day 48)

FIRST BATH TODAY!!! Oh my goodness!! How nerve racking, exciting and *exhilarating* all at the same time!! You LOVED it! You floated there and kicked your little legs and didn't cry once – until we took you out! But I don't think I will try it by myself – I don't want to drown you or drop you on the floor on the way out of the bath!!

5/4/13 (Day 52)

Came back from a quick trip home to see your daddy to find you back on LoFlo and with an IV in your little arm. They are getting ready in case you need an emergency blood transfusion. All you are doing now is sleeping and you rarely wake up anymore – I haven't seen your gorgeous smile now for days. All I want is for you to be healthy and bright-eyed again. And they have put your gavage tube back in through your mouth instead of through your nose – which you HATE. It makes you gag and dry reach. It's horrible to watch – it's like torture. But they reckon they can't have the gavage tube AND the LoFlo in your nose at the same time. Funny? – I'm sure you did before.

And you are also now back on your daily caffeine.

7/4/13 (Day 54)

Your IV line and LoFlo were removed today – they decided (again!) not to do a blood transfusion just yet. And your gavage tube is back in through your nose. You seem SO MUCH happier now. I reckon the IV, LoFlo and mouth tube was making you depressed. You are even waking up again for short periods of time instead of lying there like you are comatose. It broke my heart to see you like that. They will check your haemoglobin levels again in the morning to see where it's at. You pulled your gavage tube out AGAIN this morning! Cheeky!! That's twice two days ago when it was in through your mouth, and once today just after they put it back in through your nose.

That seems to be ANOTHER one of your pet hates – Gavage tubes!!

9/4/13 (Day 56)

You had your hearing test done today. It had to be done while you were asleep, so the lady tried to do it while I was having a cuddle with you. But it was too noisy in the bay with all the machines around you beeping and going off – so we were taken to a quiet room. And as you are not allowed to carry a baby through the Neo Unit, we were wheeled through on the breastfeeding chair!! Beep Beep!!! You passed the test – it appears you DO INDEED have ears! But seriously, it proves that there is proper function between brain waves and the ears, apparently. We had to give you another bath afterwards – the little ear muff things they used got stuck to your hair, so we had to soak them off.

12.4.13 (Day 59)

Crap! Doc S. ordered for your cardiac monitoring to come off this morning during his rounds. But your nurses agreed after he had gone NOT to take you off it just yet, as you only ceased your caffeine again yesterday and its protocol to keep cardiac monitoring on for a few days once they stop the caffeine. Plus, your first lot of needles are coming up in a couple of days – and you have to be on cardiac monitoring for that for twenty-four hours after.

14/4/13 (Day 61)

You had your two-month immunisations today. I was beside myself with worry, after they told me all the possible side effects you might have. But you didn't even get a temp. I couldn't bring myself to be there when they did it, so I waited in the Parent Room again like a big old sook. I can't stand to see pain inflicted on you.

15/4/13 (Day 62)

Aaaaaaargh!! Doc S. took your Cardiac leads off this morning on rounds – just pulled them off and told the nurse to turn off the monitor. I almost fell off my stool! I wasn't ready for that to happen yet – it was my safety net. I sit here day in, day out, and watch the numbers do their thing on the monitor, and from that I can see what your heart and resp. are doing. Now I have nothing to watch except for your sats monitor that is attached to the oximeter on your foot. But it is progress, which is a GOOD thing!

20/4/13 (Day 67)

We are now residents of the Satellite Nursery!! Upgrade!! I'm not too sure how I feel about it – yes, it's another positive step in the right direction and a step closer to going home – but this nursery is less "clinical," much quieter and a lot more "laid back" than the NNU. There are two nurses to eight babies up here, so less attention to each baby. You are the only baby up here still on the oximeter monitor – and when it goes off, meaning you are having a desat; the nurses ignore it most times. I have to keep telling them so they chart it down. But this Nursery has a huge window that lets in the sunshine – something the NNU doesn't have. And I am allowed to wheel you out of the nursery up here and out into the corridor to the little lounge area for some quiet "us" time. That's a bit special.

22/4/13 (Day 69)

Well, finally you are getting your blood transfusion today. It has only taken them 4.5 weeks to decide to do it. The nurses said we would have had our breastfeeding established by now if you had of had the energy to suck – but it was all just too tiring for you with such a low haemoglobin level. Ward Senior put her foot down and told Doc on rounds this morning that it needs to be done. They should have done this back when they first knew about it. So – we made it up to the Satellite Nursery, now we have to go back to the NSCU for the blood transfusion and you have to go back on cardiac monitoring while it happens. Doc S. says it will "wake you up" – so I am half expecting to come in tomorrow and see you crawling around on the floor!

(Pm) I sat with you throughout the transfusion; and it was one muck up after another.

I was ready to bop someone. Firstly, after they bought you back from putting in the IV lines, I noticed the backs of both your little hands were bruised. They had tried to put the line in (in) one hand – two or three times – but failed, so then they tried it on the other hand a couple times until they succeeded. Next, after the transfusion started, they noticed your IV line had a kink in it. Then, after they fixed that, the nurse forgot to turn the little tap thingy back on (on) the machine that leads to your IV drip – and the blood went back into the bag instead of into YOU! So what should have only taken about four hours, ended up taking six. You were so hungry and wriggly by the end, but I couldn't feed you because apparently feeding during a blood transfusion can lead to NECS? I was so relieved when it was over.

23/4/13 (Day 70)

Came in early this morning to find you with lovely rosy red cheeks!! What a difference. Your nurse suggested I offer you a breastfeed – you took to it like a piranha! Success!!! Was told you pulled out your IV overnight. Naughty Boy! But I can't say I blame you. I know those cannula things hurt like hell if you bump them, *and* to have one in YOUR tiny little arm must be so very painful. You had another successful breastfeed this evening. Way to go!! Nurse keeps asking me if I will allow them to bottle feed you instead of gavage when I am not here (overnight) to breastfeed you, but I said NO – not after the choking episode you had upstairs in the Satellite Nursery last week where you turned blue. That was just too scary. I thought you were going to die on me in my arms …

24/4/13 (Day 71)

Third eye test – all CLEAR!! No ROP!!!!! No more eye tests now until your follow up visit at nine months. Nasty things.

10/5/13 (Day 87)

Lots has happened since my last entry; some not so good so will remain unwritten.

Long and short of it: we are back up in the Satellite Nursery again, and you have NO leads or monitoring of any kind now. Just a bare baby. The day they took off your oximeter monitor, I rang your nurse overnight to make sure you were still breathing!

I have decided I'm not too sure about a certain doctor in particular – who I won't name – after what he did to you when he took out your gavage tube and made you practically starve for a day to try and force you to breastfeed properly. That was just cruel. I understand that unless they TRY these things, they won't know whether you are ready yet or not, but I TOLD him you weren't ready to have it out yet, that you had only JUST started breastfeeding after your transfusion. But he wouldn't listen!! He said it would teach you how to suck for your feeds faster. I was in tears all day that day. I have never seen a baby chuck such a tantrum, and all because you were beside yourself with hunger but couldn't quite get it together enough to suck for it.

The nurses were concerned the transfusion wasn't done in time and that we had lost that 'window' of opportunity for you to learn to suck swallow/breathe.

I had to give you back to the nurse at one stage; I just couldn't deal with the situation. I felt so bad for you, and so very angry at the whole situation. And AGAIN, I felt useless, that I wasn't able to placate or console you.

(Pm). Just been told you have been drafted for a back transfer to Mount Gambier Hospital

Next week; so they are doing last minute discharge checks – Physio, ECG, Cranial Ultrasound, Speech Path. The prospect of leaving here is daunting yet exciting. I don't know if I am ready to leave or not. I am so scared something will happen to you back home, or you will suddenly go backwards like you have been doing periodically up until now.

Plus, you still don't know how to breastfeed properly yet, and you still aren't pooing on your own without help.

12/5/13 (Day 89)

Mother's Day!! Came in this morning to find a beautiful card from you to me, complete with your little hand print inside. No wonder the nurses kicked me out at 2am!!! They wanted to get all the cards written and stamped by each baby for each mum; in between the usual feeds, meds and weighs. I bet they were cursing me for staying so late!!

Then, some of the mummies from the Neo support group "Women Who Have Been There" came through and gave every mum a gift bag of goodies and a cup cake. How spoilt are we?! And how nice of them!! Red Velvet! Washed down with a cuppa. You can enjoy that through my milk, later...

Mmmmmm!

Just been told our transfer has been delayed; something to do with Medstar and flights. I was apprehensive about a transfer, but after being told that – I feel really depressed and upset. Deep down, I must have wanted to go home after all.

13/5/13 (Day 90)

HOLY CRAP!! It's all happening!! On rounds this morning Doc S said, "This mum needs to be with her baby – make it happen" ". So Ward Senior has been on the phone, and flights have been booked for transfer TOMORROW!! Plus, Doc S wants us to "room in" tonight; to give you and me some private time alone before we go back to the Mount Gambier Hospital. So I have to race back to the flat and pack up all my stuff. Panic! Excitement! Anxious! Scared!

(Pm). Sitting in our Rooming In room, head is literally buzzing. It's deathly quiet in here. So quiet, it's loud. It took me two hours to pack all my stuff from the flat and tidy up!! Didn't know I had accumulated so much stuff over the past thirteen weeks. Thought I was going to need a trailer! Now we are alone. Just you and me. It's like a motel room, only inside the hospital. It's got two single beds, a table and chairs and a small lounge chair. Outside our door is a share facility kitchen/shower/toilet with the other rooming in room right next door to us.

I don't know what to do now. I have just been sitting here, watching you sleep in your crib. It feels so foreign. No nurses.

No noise from machines or other babies crying. I know I should be sleeping, I have a long drive ahead of me in the morning. But I just keep watching you to make sure you are breathing. There is a phone in here that is linked direct to the NNU if I need assistance. And I have to take you down there overnight for a check and weigh. I can't believe, after ninety days; we are finally ALONE together, just the two of us. It's so surreal. I am trying to breastfeed you as much as possible, because your gavage tube was removed this morning; mostly due to you half pulling it out and they were going to have to put a new one in anyway. They have given me some bottles of your milk, but I don't want to use them and risk you choking again – especially seeing as there isn't a nurse in here to help if you do! OMG – I can't get my head around the fact, WE ARE GOING HOME TO MOUNT GAMBIER TOMORROW!!!!!

14/5/13 (Day 91)

I knew this all along in advance, but I still think it's so unfair that I am not allowed to travel with you back on the plane and I have to drive myself back – which means I have to leave you YET AGAIN in the NNU. I can't stop crying. I don't want to be separated from you again. Not after having you to myself all night last night like a normal mum and baby. And, we don't know what TIME Medstar will be collecting you for the flight home today. I may beat you there, I may not. I may get home and have to wait for YOU to arrive. But, we will be together again very soon, my Lil' Man.

And then we can finally begin our life together: You, me and your daddy, as a *family* – as was meant to be. XXXXXXXXX

CHAPTER NINE

I won't lie to you. Giving birth prematurely and subsequently having that baby living In a Neo ward indefinitely for months on end is NOT easy. And you have to find new strength EACH day from resources you never knew you had – and you DO, because you have a little life that depends on you to do so. And that old cliché "unless you have been there, you won't understand?" It is SO true. It's easy to be on the outside looking in, hearing about someone else's baby, and the daily adversities that they face.

But to have to personally LIVE it, SEE it, HEAR it and BREATHE it, day in day out for an undetermined length of time… it changes you, for both better and for worse, but one thing it DOES do to you is give you a stronger sense of life meaning, a higher appreciation of the battle these little miracle babies face – and you tend not to take anything for granted anymore, because you NOW KNOW the extraordinary effort such a fragile existence hinges on.

The *journey* you just took with me, ultimately, as I mentioned at the very start; changed my *life*. What you just read wasn't some fanciful, whimsical made up fable.

It was my sad and deplorable existence for a long ninety-one days, while the rest of my life was suspended in time. I can't vouch for other Premmie Mum's, but I know the whole ordeal took its toll on me and affected ME profoundly, every day, in everything I did and in every decision I made; in even the most innocent of ways.

I strongly believe, the way I viewed things after our long Neo stay was directly predicated by what I lived and breathed and saw on a daily basis inside those Neonatal walls. You can't witness all those things without being mentally scarred from it.

For a start – I practised what is regarded to be THE cardinal sin of Parenting 101 ... I co – slept with my baby.

I knew it wasn't recommended due to the risk of SIDS, and it was in complete contradiction to every other cautious way I was caring for my son. It was part of the Baby Resus course content I took while we were still in the Neo. Pages and pages of reasons why NOT to sleep with your baby. And just because I am admitting I did it – and am STILL doing it – does NOT mean I am advocating the practice.

But I needed it: needed the closeness, needed to further cement our bond.

I had a lot of cuddle time to make up for. The anguished memories of him lying in his crib at night in the Neo, alone, for ninety long nights, without my love and warmth to comfort him was insurmountable. So I learnt to sleep propped upright with my baby on my chest. Then, as he got older and bigger, I learnt to sleep without a pillow on the bed. My decision to co-sleep was a calculated risk, but I felt it was rationally justified. Again, I am not advocating the practice. It was MY personal choice. As with anything you decide in relation to your child – the way you choose to bring them up and the parenting practices you adopt whilst doing so is solely YOUR choice because it works for YOU. It should not be a contentious issue.

I know there are guidelines and recommendations, but I strongly believe there is no "right" or wrong way. No one else's opinion matters if you are comfortable in what you are doing, and have the informed conviction to stand by what you do, and take the necessary precautions.

As a first-time mother, it could be forgiven that I was out of my depth. Babies, and indeed Prems, don't come with a parenting manual or handbook. But factoring in both of these, loaded with a Neo experience combined, paved the way for something more insidious. And you will easily be able to see the direct correlation between my Neo journey and my Postnatal Depression. Having said that, I am not saying ALL Mum's who have a prem baby and a Neo journey will end up with Postnatal Depression.

I'm just saying I believe this was true in MY case. As strong as I thought I was, Post-Neo I just fell to pieces.

I know babies, in general, are time-wasters – just like a litter of puppies, you can sit and watch them all day and achieve little else, which is exactly what I did, daily, for hours on end for the first few months after coming home from hospital. But I did it for a different reason than out of fascinated awe. I did it out of sheer terror.

I would study him intently, wondering if he was having a brady, a desat or apnoea; counting his heart and respiration rate. I would try to decide if his breathing was normal or recessive, or if his pallour was his usual colour. It was the internal things I could not see, that kept me anxiously preoccupied. I knew the doctors wouldn't have released him if he was still at risk, but at the same time, I was petrified that he would 'crash' on me like he used to in the Neo. At least back there, the cardio machines would alarm to alert the nurses. At home, I didn't have that technological safety net. I had to use my own uneducated and untried judgement.

I was worried sick that I might miss some small vital sign of his health beginning to deteriorate that I became obsessed with over the top monitoring; Charting his Obs every hour just like in the Neo, following by example just as I had seen his healthcare providers do.

Not dispassionately, not indifferently, and certainly not in a detached manner devoid of love for my son. Quite the opposite – I loved him so fiercely that I felt I had to be on high alert 24/7 to protect him at all costs. He'd already been through so much as a direct result of my body failing to carry him to Term; and I was now feverishly determined I wouldn't fail him again in ANY way. I felt I couldn't afford to be complacent, not for one second; and that I couldn't indulge in the blind joys of motherhood because I had to put my baby's health above all else. But in my quest to prove my worth and competence as a mother and care provider, coupled with my increasing pre-occupation of my son's well-being, I forgot to appreciate and enjoy my precious bundle for what he was. The months flew by, and suddenly, I had a somewhat independent toddler in his place. I now deeply regret the unnecessary time I wasted agonising over the state of his health. Even my doctor asked me on more than one occasion how much longer I was going to record every little thing concerning my son. I literally carried the clipboard with the chart sheet with me when I left the house, complete with pen and thermometer. It was MY way of taking back control of my life. But one day I suddenly realised my baby was no longer the helpless baby I was so used to seeing; and once again, I felt ripped off (of) another maternal experience. First had been my pregnancy, cut short way before I had the opportunity to fully savour its joys, of which I personally consider pregnancy the ultimate rite of passage into motherhood, and I feel like I missed something vitally important by not seeing it through to the end.

And seemingly, in the blink of an eye, the swaddling and kangaroo cuddles and Bassinette were gone too.

If there is one piece of advice I would give to new Premmie mums just discharged from the Neo, it would be: Don't deny yourself of this incredible bundle of joy. You have just been through hell and back with your baby, watching from the side-lines instead of being the hands-on mother you so desperately wanted to be – so ENJOY your baby while he or she is still so, because that stage is fleeting and over way too quickly. And too much of it is already lost from your time spent in the NICU.

It wasn't just the 'babyhood' I felt I missed due to my ministrations as a direct result of coming fresh out of the Neonatal Unit. It also prevented me from embracing the NEXT few phases of my child's development – sitting up, crawling and moving onto solids. In my mind, I still had to keep him wrapped in cotton wool for his own protection. To ME, he was still so fragile. Instead of letting him explore his world and find himself, I kept him in his pram and pushed him throughout the house in it wherever I went. At 12 months old (9 months corrected age), he still wasn't sitting up an-assisted. It wasn't until our *first follow-up* visit back at Flinders that I realised how much I was holding him back as a direct result of my own fears and angst.

We were looking at possibly seeing a child physio if things didn't start progressing, and a speech pathologist for his eating aversion due to me not giving him the opportunity to move on to solids. I had been SO paranoid that he would choke and literally die in front of me that I had delayed the introduction of textured foods to the point that it was fast becoming to HIS detriment. My obsessions about his health and well-being had ended up inadvertently creating problems when there otherwise wouldn't have been any. We were already looking at possible development delays due to his gestation, and it was now a fine line as to WHAT was the cause of him being 'behind' at this age.

So as hard as it was for me, I had to 'let go' a little and let him do his own thing.

And seemingly, in no time, he was moving forward in leaps and bounds.

At 12.5 months old (9.5 months corrected age), he could sit up. By 14 months (11 months corrected age), he was crawling. And by 16 months (13 months corrected age), he was walking. By 17 months (14 months corrected), he was well onto solid foods ... including meats. But even though we were progressing, it was still a lot of effort that left me in tears every day. We still even had a few feeding issues at 21 months old (18 months corrected age).

It took a while, and it was a stressful time for me, but once it was pointed out to me that I was the cause of him not achieving the targeted milestones, I had to take a serious look at myself and what I was doing. My over protecting him was, in fact, oppressing him. His learning potential and motor skill growth were being severely suppressed.

You might be wondering, WHAT I was just referring to by the mention of "Corrected Age," just now?

It took ME a while to get a handle on it, but when talking about the AGE of a prem baby, you will more often than not hear TWO ages – Firstly, their ACTUAL age, followed by the age they WOULD HAVE BEEN if they had been born on their Due Date; which is referred to as their CORRECTED AGE.

For example, I just talked about my son crawling at 14mths old (11 months corrected).

He was BORN in February 2013, but wasn't DUE until May 2013.

This might seem confusing to some people, but it is important due to the fact that a prem baby grows and develops according to their CORRECTED AGE (because TECHNICALLY, they were born before they had finished growing and maturing).

So while you may look at a prem baby of actual age – in REALITY, developmentally wise, they are still only at the stage of their GESTATIONAL age corrected. So for MY son, at whatever age he was, you'd take OFF 3 months – to allow for his gestational prematurity. Some parents even allow their premmies to have TWO birthdays …one for their actual age, and then another for when they were actually due to have been born. I myself just go by my son's ACTUAL birthdate; because for ME, to celebrate it twice would feel too much like a slap in the face as a crude reminder of my physical failure – but I also fully understand and respect why others do it differently.

So WHEN do prems STOP being referred to AS a prem, you might ask? Good question. According to the research, most preterm infants catch up in body Growth by three years of age. Very low birth weight (less than 1500gm at birth)

Infants will take longer to reach their growth weight potential. While at three years of age 50% of small for gestational age (SGA) babies are below normal growth, most of these catch up by seven to eight years of age.

At age 20 mths/17 Corrected age, my son weighed 10.3kg. I knew of other prems that weighed this at 9mths of age. I also knew of older prems that weighed around this at about 2.5 years of age, which only further reinforces the fact that each baby is unique and cannot be compared – at ANY time – to another. So don't despair or be despondent if your premmie isn't following any particular trend. They are doing the best that their little bodies are capable of and will get there in their own time. It isn't a race or a contest.

So it is MY understanding that by eight years of age, for all intents and purposes, they should have hit all their developmental milestones, and would be being assisted in the areas found to be lacking in. By age eight, most families of premmies would finally be starting to get their lives back.

Which flows nicely onto this next subject.

Frustratingly, DISCHARGE from the Neonatal Ward and hospital isn't where it ends for a Prem. I alluded not so long ago to our first Follow Up visit back at Flinders…

Regular Follow-up Medical and Growth & Development visits in Adelaide are required so progress can be monitored – and intervention can be applied – at the earliest possible sign of a problem.

These visits include: Full Medicals, Ongoing Eye Checks, Hearing Tests, Gross Motor Skill Development Assessments, appointments with a Physio and Speech Pathologist etc., etc.

The LENGTH of the Follow-up Program varies from three years of age to eight years of age, dependant of the following criteria: (at least, this is applicable for the Flinder's Neonatal Unit Follow-Up Program … Other hospitals may differ.)

* ALL babies born at less than 32 weeks and/or less than 1500gm will have these follow-up appointments until the age of 3.

* Babies born at less than 30 weeks and or less than 1250gm will continue having Follow-ups until age 5.

* And babies born at 28 weeks and under and /or less than 1000gm have THEIR Follow-ups extended to 8 yrs of age.

(Also included in the Follow-up Program are babies deemed High Risk at birth (irrelevant of their birth gestation) IE: Those with Hypoxia, or born not initially breathing at all.)

When we were sent an appointment card in the mail a couple months before the scheduled time for our first Follow-up G&D visit, I was so stressed. All I could think about was having to watch my son be subjected to all these invasive tests, and I could already hear him screaming in protest and pain. They used to tell us that as little babies, they wouldn't remember their time in the Neo, and the procedures they underwent. But as a nearly 12 month old, I was petrified for him. He would certainly remember it THIS time!

On the drive up to Adelaide, I felt sick and was so protective of Aidan that I sat in the back next to him the whole way while my Dad drove. He had to know, I was there for him. If he had to go through all that all over again – I was right there by his side.

I was also physically nauseous at the thought of going back to the Neo itself. Walking those corridors. Riding those lifts. Smelling that distinct scent. Hearing the multitude of machines as they chorused and alerted the nurses of what was happening with each and every baby.

But on the day, after all the previous angst and working myself up over it; it was all for nought. Surprisingly, walking through the hospital was more nostalgic than anything, and entering the doors of the Neonatal Unit wasn't nearly as bad as I had been thinking it would be. I did have tears in my eyes, but the feeling that accompanied them was like exhaling after holding your breath for so long. Relief. In a way, it was like coming home.

Some of the nurses came out to the Parent Room to greet us and fuss over Aidan, and then we were taken through the unit to see all the other nurses so they could see Aidan and marvel at how he had grown since his birth.

They admit they don't recognise the baby/child, because they look so different to when they were patients… But they remember the mums (I don't know if that is a good remark or not!), and most of them remembered ME, because of the cupcakes I used to bake them.

And the tests were nothing more than observations, really. There was no bloodletting.

There were no tears. Weight and height measurements were taken, a listen to his heart and lungs with a stethoscope, discussions about his health since discharge; and then the Physio played on the floor with him with some toys to see what his minor and gross motor skills were developing like. The eye test was the main procedure I was worried about – I was NOT relishing having to sit and watch THAT … But again, I had worked myself up unnecessarily because it was all non-invasive this time round. I was so pent up and worried sick about the whole day that when our last appointment was over, I nearly collapsed in emotional exhaustion. And it was at THAT point, that all I wanted was to get out of the hospital and on the road back to home.

I had a fair bit to think about on the long drive back to Mt Gambier. I had left Flinders this day feeling thoroughly demoralised. It was at this first visit back to Flinders that I learned my son wasn't hitting the projected 'age specific' milestones. I had thought we had been doing so well, so it was quite distressful to hear otherwise. I had tortured thoughts of what it might mean for his future, and once again – I was blaming myself. If only I'd done things differently.

So having a Prem isn't JUST a deviation and adjustment from "the norm" at birth, – it's ongoing for quite a few years to come AFTER that; and a drain on the hip pocket and an emotional strain alike. It sometimes gets to the point where you think – Where does it end??? You just want a normal lifestyle and to enjoy your family, without all the added inconvenience, stress, worry and interference.

And it extends way beyond the physical and visual implications related to the consequences of being born premature. It's also unforeseen things, like (for want of an example), what condition your child's TEETH will be in once their adult teeth start coming down at 6 – 8 years of age.

The teeth (the full set of twenty) are formed in the gums whilst your baby is still in-utero, and any interference at this important stage of foetal development (i.e. – birth before Term) can result in damaged teeth as their young pearly whites emerge.

Sometimes you can see early evidence of this from their baby teeth by way of lack of enamel …Teeth that appear 'stained' or 'dirty'. But for many, it is yet another waiting game. This damage can sometimes spill over to their adult teeth as well.

So babies born prematurely affects a lot more aspects of their future lives than most realise. For some prems, the health implications are ongoing and relentless. Having prem babies is a fact of life, something that is out of our control, but until it happens to YOU, you don't fully understand the hardships and the emotional rollercoaster that goes with it.

Which now brings me back to the main reason for writing this book:

POSTNATAL DEPRESSION.

Too many people have the wrong impression of what PND actually is, and about how it affects women that are suffering from it. And THAT stereotypical misnomer needs to be addressed and corrected. Women suffering from it need to be empowered with the knowledge that they are not alone in what they are going through – and to not be afraid to seek help to manage it and overcome it. If you are diagnosed with Postnatal

Depression, it does not mean you are weak. That is not the reason you have it. Women of strong constitution also find themselves at the mercy of PND. All women from every age, race, colour and creed suffer from it. It doesn't care about your social status, or socio-economic prestige – it's indiscriminate and strikes at random.

Pride, embarrassment and fear are very real reasons why women don't want to admit they are struggling and need help – but take it from someone who knows first-hand what it feels like to be drowning in the abyss of despair: You may THINK you have it under control and can get through it on your own, but the only person you are kidding is yourself. When you are wrapped up in your own little world, it is all too easy to tell yourself that everything is okay and that it's just a 'phase' you are going through. But it won't just 'go away' if you try and ignore it. It will fester. It will consume you. It will bring you to your knees, and sometimes it will do just that, in spectacular fashion.

I was diagnosed with PND about three months after we were discharged from Flinders.

I was lonely – so very, very lonely; especially after being up in Adelaide by myself for thirteen weeks. But bizarrely, I didn't want to see anyone. I shut myself in my house and didn't venture out except for the weekly grocery shop. And as I previously mentioned – even with that came huge obstacles for me. It was like I forgot how to function in public; like I was walking around with a bag on my head. I lost all my confidence. I second guessed my ability to do anything and everything, especially if I was by myself.

I was ALWAYS in tears; I had no control over them. I would cry along with my son when he cried, but I would still be crying long after he had stopped. I would cry in confusion and frustration. I would cry in desperation. I would cry with the overwhelming burden of having someone rely solely on ME for their every want and need – as I struggled to distinguish exactly WHAT those needs were. I would cry in empathy at the slightest hint of discord. I would cry in relief. I couldn't believe how many tears one person could have. I would get differing stares from strangers if I went out in public, because I just couldn't control my teary episodes. My eyes were perpetually red and puffy.

Some people would give me a kind, tentative, sympathetic smile; while others would just blatantly stare and silently condemn and judge. I would be eating my tea and realise, yet again, that I had tears pouring down my cheeks. My husband would ask me: "What's wrong"? And I couldn't tell him, because I didn't know! All I knew was, I felt this unexplained and inexplicable, incredible sadness.

In frustration, my husband would often tell me that I should be feeling grateful and lucky for the miracle son we had, and reminded me that the outcome could have very well gone the other way and that I could have come home empty-handed like a lot of other Neo mum's do – which only served to make me feel MORE guilty and ashamed for everything I was feeling.

I berated myself constantly .... How could I have this blessed little baby and *yet* still feel so totally bereft? Was I THAT ungrateful and selfish?? What the hell was WRONG with me???

My poor suffering husband – God Bless him – he was always there for me, but as much as he thought he was being supportive, even HE didn't understand what it was that I felt.

In HIS opinion, our Neo journey had ended and we were home – end of story. Move on.

He couldn't understand my feelings of loss and grief, because in his opinion – I hadn't LOST anything. He didn't understand the unexplained incredible sadness I was feeling.

He didn't understand the self-loathing and resentment and the emptiness. He would often say, "Just think of how you would be feeling right now if Aidan had died and you'd come home without him?" or "You should be grateful and happy he's even here at all." Sometimes, in sheer frustration, he would lash out if I was having a "moment," and he'd tell me to, "Go take a pill and chill." He truly DID try hard to comprehend my depressive state, but even HE admits it's something he just didn't 'get'. Sometimes, witnessing me have a complete meltdown was so disturbing for him, that he had to leave the house. The fact that he didn't understand what I was feeling meant he felt at a loss as to how to comfort me. And I guess that in turn made HIM feel emasculated. And if that's coming from someone who had, in essence, travelled the journey WITH me – what hope does someone ELSE have of understanding it, unless they have experienced it for themselves?

I felt like a HUGE failure – for not being able to carry my baby to Term. And I thoroughly hated myself for what Aidan had (had) to go through as a direct result of my physical ineptness. On more than one occasion, I admit – I wanted to feel some form of hurt; as in PHYSICAL pain, as my penance for what Aidan had suffered through. I felt like I deserved it. I felt it was only fair.

On the days where it all just got too much for me, and I was being driven crazy by the white noise in my head; I wanted so badly to smack myself hard across the face, to feel that sting – to feel ANYTHING, really. But instead, I would just sit there, hands clenched into fists so tight that my fingernails would be driven so far into the skin on my palms that they would almost bleed, and hold my breath until the inside of my head went black and the buzzing stopped.

I started to think maybe my body had been trying to tell me that I shouldn't have been a "mum" in the first place. That I had no business taking on that role. That I wasn't good enough. I truly felt like I didn't deserve to be happy.

Some days I felt like I couldn't even breathe – like someone had their hands around my throat. On the outside I looked fine, but majority of the time, my whole body just seemed to buzz. I felt on edge and 'electrified'; like a rubber band stretched to its limit and about to snap; like I was on a hysterical or euphoric high but at the same time, I had no energy or desire to do anything. I always felt drained and lethargic. Which sounds absurd and totally contradictory, I know – but I bet there are a lot of mums out there who can relate to what I've just described. It's the insidious physical manifestation of depression. It silently saps you of everyday happiness.

Everything loses its appeal. Where you once found enjoyment you now have an empty void. And even though your mind is racing a million miles an hour, you feel physically heavy and exhausted. You have overwhelming, unexplained feelings of incredible sadness and a deep emptiness that you just can't shake. You feel a constant dread in the pit of your stomach that you just can't explain and which never seems to go away.

You go about your daily business on pure auto-pilot, doing things by rote. All your senses and emotions are heightened and over exaggerated, but you are helpless to control them. I knew I was becoming increasingly snappy and over-sensitive. It was like having an out of body experience. I could feel it happening, could even hear myself speak the words – but I couldn't stop it. My poor husband would make a general comment and I would get irrational and all bent out of shape. I always took his comments as personal attacks and felt like he was pointing out how useless I was. If he so much as tried to help with a household chore, I took it as his disapproving way of telling me I wasn't coping or keeping up. I was on the defensive, 24/7. I just couldn't help it. I started to resent his succour, because it only served to make me feel even MORE superfluous. Everything he said felt patronising. It's no fun feeling like everything you do is wrong or not good enough. And it's not nice when you have convinced yourself that everyone is against you. Or worse still – completely ambivalent to what you are going through. Believe me when I say, you can be in a crowded room, yet still feel desperately alone. My proprietary morale hit rock bottom.

In my misery, as I said, I put on 15 kgs. And the antibiosis of that was, I felt like I had lost my sexual attractiveness and hence, I completely lost my libido. I felt repulsed at what had become of my body. I didn't want my husband to have to be subjected to it. And I also felt extremely vulnerable, after having my husband witness our child's birth. For him to have seen what happens in childbirth – it left me feeling dirty and exposed. I truly felt he would never look at me the same way again.

I didn't blame my pregnancy for the change – I blamed myself. And I still felt like I had no control over anything. I felt like I had lost my anonymity. It dawned on me that I didn't know who I WAS anymore…

My PND fed off my self-inflicted OCD, and vice versa. My OCD became 'OTT' (over the top). I became ultra-paranoid and anxious about germs and bugs – I was petrified that Aidan would end up back in hospital. The meaning of the word "GERM" took on a whole new definition for me. Fresh out of the sanitised refuge of the Neo, the enormity of how disastrous the consequences of a possible bacterial invasion could really be suddenly turned me into my own worst enemy. If someone so much as touched him, I would have a panic attack and still be anxious about it hours later; agonising as to if he was going to get sick – and then panicking as to HOW sick.

Like I said earlier on, in my mind's eye I could literally SEE the bugs and germs marching off of people's hands and onto my baby. Like the caricature germs on TV ads – only the ones I saw weren't all cutesy; I saw these ones as being much nastier with fangs and horns and warts because I now knew how much havoc they could cause.

It frustrated me that every person that saw Aidan always felt the necessity to have to touch his face and cheeks. Literally, the first place they zeroed in on was the face and cheeks – and sometimes even brushed their fingers over his lips.

I don't know how many times I got physically light-headed because I was so incensed and panicked whenever it happened. My son's health was on the line, yet people were totally oblivious to it. It got to the point where I was starting to avoid people, just so they couldn't get near him. I KNOW that a baby has to have exposure to germs in order to strengthen their immune systems – but in regards to a Prem baby, whose immune system is already compromised, I think it is wiser to err on the side of caution and choose your battles wisely. There is nothing to be gained by socialising your prem baby who has chronic lung disease with someone who has a raging head cold or the flu. That's just asking for trouble. Common sense should prevail, but, as we all have differing opinions about how to raise our children, it will be at the discretion of each individual parent. And I totally respect that. But when people tell me I am being ridiculous and over-cautious by keeping my baby in confinement, I take offence to that and get quite angry. They have not seen what I saw. They weren't the ones who had to keep a tenuous cribside vigil each day for the first three months of their baby's life.

I wouldn't even go into my bird aviaries to feed my birds without showering afterwards, or at the very least, changing every piece of my clothing. I was worried that if any of my birds had Air Sac Mite that I might take it back to Aidan. He already had chronic lung disease as a legacy of being prem, and I didn't want to risk him catching anything that might potentially make his breathing worse. Which just goes to show HOW paranoid and over the top careful I really was – because Air Sac Mite is NOT a zoonotic disease.

And I KNEW that from the animal Husbandry courses I had taken over the years.

Yet, I was still zealously cautious. I just couldn't help it.

And I just continued to feel so incredibly sad. The weight of the sadness was the worst. The only joy I felt was when I was physically holding Aidan, yet even then, I still felt hopelessly lost. I couldn't stop thinking about what we'd been through in the Neo, about what I'd seen.

It just kept replaying in my mind, over and over and over...

And if I saw a pregnant woman in public or on TV, I got uncharacteristically jealous of the fact THEY were still pregnant. I felt a deep-seated solicitousness I can't quite explain. Seeing other pregnant women only highlighted my failure to carry my own baby, which made me think unfair and unsavoury thoughts, and I hated myself all more for it. I certainly didn't wish them any ill will, but I so desperately wanted what they still had – a blossomed baby bump. The pangs of wistfulness and longing were physically painful.

I was consumed with needing to find a reason for why it happened, to lay the blame somewhere else but with me. I was angry. I had done everything right. And yet STILL, it had all gone so wrong. I continued to trawl the Premmie Support pages on Facebook and scour the internet on my laptop daily looking for company, comradery – and answers. It wasn't just that I WANTED answers … I NEEDED answers.

Everything that had happened and everything that I went through has irrevocably changed my whole life. Even NOW, I am still consumed with the why.

(Going back) to the initial suggestion that I was suffering from PND came from my CAFHS nurse on one of their routine home visits, but I ignored it because I was scared.

It terrified me to think that if I was "labelled" with PND, that someone would come and take my baby off me.

I had (had) my baby taken off me at birth, and then I wasn't able to be a proper mum to my baby for three whole months after that. I had spent ninety nights without my infant by my side; ninety nights where my arms and his waiting crib had remained empty and cold. I did not want to tempt a fate I knew would send me right over the edge. I vowed to keep it to myself and battle on.

But I was becoming increasingly depressed and anxious, so after several visits – and constant reassurance that even in the worst case scenarios (because they strive to keep mother and baby together where possible), that no-one would take my precious baby – I agreed I would go and see my doctor.

That first initial visit with my GP was intensely emotional. Once I had accepted the fact I was indeed 'broken', the floodgates were opened and I was relieved she was there for what I saw as my salvation. She was going to make things right again.

But even after acknowledging my condition, at first, I declined any sort of help that my doctor suggested. I was convinced that just by readily embracing the fact that I HAD Postnatal Depression, meant I could get over it on my own. I have always been the type of person to sort out my own problems, and I truly believed I could sort THIS out by myself too – but after a couple more months of continual mini meltdowns, I finally accepted that I COULDN'T deal with it by myself, and I went back and sought further help.

I was referred to a Counsellor to start with, followed by a script for anti-depressants.

My counsellor said I was suffering from what she called "Survivors Guilt"; of having been through the emotional trauma of a Neo Journey and come out the other side; but not being able to let it go, and feeling guilty that I came home with a healthy baby when there are others who aren't so lucky ... and, that I was most likely to also be suffering from Post-Traumatic Stress Syndrome as a direct result OF our Neo Journey.

Talking about it all and getting things into perspective really helped. Being told that, however irrational my warped way of thinking may seem – that it WAS a legitimate coping mechanism for everything that I had been through and was feeling. THAT verbal validation gave me the silent permission to better understand and accept what it was that I was feeling; and even though I still have my down days, seeking help was the best thing I did because I am now in a much better place because of it.

There are still times and events that really get me down and trigger manic episodes – such as my son's birthdays.

It's confusing, because the whole goal is to see them grow up and thrive, and when they are, you feel inexplicitly saddened by it. I do believe that a lengthy Neonatal stay is what makes us want to hang onto their infancy for as long as possible.

And when my son decided it was time to wean himself from breastfeeding at 17.5 mths (14.5 mths corrected age), that was an especially sad time for me. I felt Rejected, like this was HIS revenge. I felt, again, like a failure – especially when he came down ill two weeks after weaning with Viral Bronchiolitis, and I found out that there is evidence that breastfeeding provides some protection against it. I mentally tortured myself that once AGAIN, it was MY fault he was now sick. I should have started expressing as soon as he showed signs of refusing the breast, to prolong the benefits of the goodness of Mummy's milk in his diet; so I tried expressing after nearly a month of inactivity, if only to ply him with the antibodies in my milk to help fortify his immune compromised system, but it was all in vain. My milk supply had all but dried up. All my dogged determination to keep breastfeeding despite all my obstacles – the pain and suffering I endured from my bouts of nipple thrush and mastitis, the 'attaching' issues we had for months on end which saw me in tears every time he fed … it was all now over. Masochistically, I missed it. Nursing is such a beautiful and calming experience (when it's established correctly!). I was sorry to see it end. My days of breastfeeding were finished.

The realisation that my baby truly was no longer "a baby" was difficult for me to accept.

Watching certain things on TV or seeing something baby/premmie related on Facebook still affects me greatly – it's like a sucker punch that leaves you winded. I am not joking when I say, after having a Neonatal experience, you are left licking your wounds for some time to come.

And some days, I just feel melancholy and have the urge to look back on photos of when my son was in the NICU; to perversely remember how it felt, if for no other reason than to further imprint how fortunate we truly were – and to fully appreciate what we truly have.

CHAPTER TEN

So where am I, mentally and emotionally, nearly two years down the track?

I will continue to blame myself for my baby being born so premature. And unless I have an unforeseen epiphany, I doubt that will ever change.

I just can't accept that a body which is fully equipped to procreate and nurture can just 'fail' for no apparent reason. I know this train of thought is a tad illogical and most assuredly unhealthy, but in the absence of a distinct medical reason, I just can't fathom any other answer for it. I failed – pure and simple. And this is a psychological dilemma I will be battling for some time to come. What makes it even worse is that I didn't even fall into any 'category' for my preterm labour. At least if I was categorised, I might be able to better deal with it. To fall into a category would have been a REASON. And if there had been a REASON, I could maybe understand and accept it. I COULD have been pPROM by default – but it would come back to that age old chestnut – Which came first (the chicken or the egg)? True pPROM is where your waters break BEFORE labour begins (Preterm Premature Rupture Of Membranes). But this usually happens because of another underlying medical issue. I don't know WHICH happened FIRST in MY case ... I was asleep at the time. The doctors just say it was spontaneous, with probable Sepsis (infection) – but nothing was confirmed. And what makes it all the MORE worse is; I had been to the Doctor THE DAY BEFORE for examination.

And was told everything was FINE. I had trusted that GP, especially seeing as this was my first pregnancy.

Just recently, after having an online discussion on a premmie site about exactly this, because I was having a particularly bad day dwelling on it (even nearly two years down the track – a REASON, a CATEGORY – a WHY – is still very important to me); another fellow premmie mum came up with an alternate 'category' which made me smile and I'd like to share it (with her permission).

Her name is Sally, and I give her full credit for this new 'category'. She said :

"Perhaps these things happen due to the phenomena of CWTSOM … translated meaning – 'Can't Wait To See Our Mum'."

Despite not placating my demons, I thought that was a beautiful sentiment.

I'm still pedantic about germs, although I am no longer maniacally wiping my son's hands over with antibacterial wipes every two seconds. I still avoid large gatherings, I don't take my son out over winter unless it's absolutely necessary, and the only "Mother's Group" I attend is the Miracle Babies Nurture Group, because they have a wellness policy. I have even started to embrace visitors with children, because I can see the sheer joy on my son's face when he is interacting with another child. I don't want to deprive him of anything, especially if he is the one to benefit.

I think it will always be in my nature to automatically blame myself when something goes wrong, especially where my son is concerned. But perhaps that's not just ME … I would think EVERY mum takes a martyring responsibility for her child's wellbeing. As mothers, I'm SURE we all wonder – at SOME point – if we could have done something BETTER, or if we are doing ENOUGH. I know I ask MY self that question at LEAST once a day! Most days I wonder if what I am doing is right or if my mothering skills are all wrong, but that is neither premmie nor PND related.

I'm sure even the most seasoned mother feels that too. I HAVE realised though, that trying to conform to someone's "idealised" way of parenting is sure to only cause much angst. What works for some, just simply does not work for others. You have to find what is right for YOU.

I do, however, constantly worry about the future global development of my son, about whether he will have any learning issues or difficulties as a result of his extreme prematurity. He SEEMS to be a very switched on and cluey little boy – but as I don't have any other kids, I don't have anything to compare his development to, and I could just be being bias in his amazing achievements to date.

Only time will tell, and in the meantime, I am just trying to enjoy him now for who and what he is – because every minute counts. The time I have lost, I won't ever get back – but I CAN make up for it from here on in by giving him 100% of myself .

And I am well aware of how lucky we have been with our son's health – both in regards with his prematurity and in his 22 months of life to date. He has only had two bouts of tonsillitis, one head cold, one lung infection (viral bronchiolitis), and recently a non-descript tummy bug that gave him the nastiest nappy rash for the first time EVER.

Not to detract from the enormity of what we went through, but these things are all pretty trivial in the scheme of things, when you consider that a lot of premmies go home still on oxygen and with their gastric feeding tubes, and have years of ongoing medical issues – so it really brings into perspective just how different each baby IS.

Our new doctor also suspects he may be asthmatic, and he can't run around for very long without coughing and getting wheezy, but that's something they can't properly diagnose until after a child turns two years old. But if asthma is the only lasting legacy of his prematurity out of the plethora of ailments he could have faced – I'll take it.

The majority of the other prem babies that were in the Neo long-term with my son have had continued health problems – and I think ALL of them have had recurrent hospital admissions periodically since their initial discharge from the Neo. That in itself makes me feel guilty for OUR good fortune, and I often wonder if we are resented because of it.

On the one hand, I am relieved it's not us, and for that I feel truly blessed, but I feel their frustrations and fears as if they were my own, because they are like extended family; and my heart aches – I wish there was something I could do for them to make it all go away. If there is one thing my whole premature birth/Neo journey has taught me, it's overwhelming empathy for others. Having been through it myself, I can now fully relate to other people's experiences; even though I know and appreciate that no two journeys are the same. As individuals, we all bring something different to the table, and when we share our story with others, we walk away with a little something we never had before. That's why I think it's beneficial to discuss our struggles and triumphs. It gives other's hope. And if there ever was a time that anyone needed hope – it's at that time when you are at your most vulnerable; as a passenger when your premmie baby is fighting for his life; one of the biggest trials and tribulations you both will ever have to fight in his entire existence.

Almost poetically, I found that when you first embark on your Neo Journey, you are scared, overwhelmed and you most definitely don't want to be there. Then, once you have been in there for a while, and immersed in its surroundings day after day after day, you still are conscious of the fact it's the last place you want to be – but you've grown to accept it. And then when you leave it, in some bizarre perverted way, you wish you were BACK in there – because it was your SAFE place. It's where you saw your baby at his worst, but it's also where you witnessed him grow and thrive.

You feel paralysed by the sudden change in dynamics, when they relinquish his care from their doctorate army, into your solitary one.

But I promise you, it gets easier. And they are only ever just a phone call away. I think it took me a good six months to fully adjust to home life after discharge. I used to sometimes even call the Neo Unit late at night when I knew they weren't overly run off their feet, to touch base with a familiar nurse and to just hear the bells and alarms in the background; even though hearing them would make me catch my breath, the sound instantly calmed me.

On a personal level, in regards to my PND – I still have days where I feel lost and alone. Some days are worse than others. I still have days where I am overcome with sudden sadness. I still cry at the drop of a hat. I let silly little things get to me. I don't know how long this will go on for or if it will ever truly go away.

I'm wondering if it will EVER get better, but then, when I look BACK at how bad I WAS, I know that in time, it DOES. But it won't ever be gone completely. I think there will always be a shadow over me.

I have 'sook sessions' at least once a week, sometimes more. And I consciously allow myself to do that, because I have come to realise that it's a form of release and – I think – a healthy part of the healing process. I see the instant concern register on my husband's face when he comes home from work and sees my puffy red eyes, and he knows straight away if my day has been good or bad. And I know that he worries that I am slipping back to where I was, But in my opinion, it's better out than in, and so long as I can muster a smile afterward, I know I'm still winning the fight.

And now, I find myself in a bit of a conundrum of late ... I swore never again would I have any more babies after what I went through with my spontaneous and unexplained Premature birth, and the subsequent Neo journey that followed.

But amazingly, around the time my son hit 18 months of age, I suddenly found myself to be entertaining the possibility of perhaps trying again, to give our son a sibling.

I don't want him to grow up alone and lonely. But I am terrified of having another prem, which THIS time the whole ordeal would be compounded even more so, because I also would have a toddler to consider as well. It wouldn't be fair on him, to be on the receiving end of a long separation away from me if I had to go to Adelaide again. And it wouldn't be realistic to take him with me, because I wouldn't be able to devote my time to him AS WELL AS to a baby in a Neo ward.

...Gosh – I could just SEE him trying to flip power switches, playing with knobs and dials, unplugging cords and get himself tangled in them, exploring cupboards and drawers and turning them inside out, and just generally getting under the nurses feet! It would be a disaster!

At my son's 18mth vaccination appointment, I told my doctor I had been considering trying again, and asked her opinion about it. She gave me a 50/50 chance of having another prem, and said that women who have prems WITHOUT cause are just that little bit MORE at risk of it happening with subsequent pregnancies, as opposed to those women who DID have a reason the first time around. At least with a known cause for it, they have a trend to follow – a 'template', if you like.

But with spontaneous preterm births, there is no history to follow, which makes it all very scary and has left me very confused and with a big decision to make. Would it be irresponsible of me to roll that dice, given the odds? Would it be foolish to tempt fate? But then, my doctor ALSO said on the flip side, I could very well carry to Term next time. The anguish is in the not knowing. But Oh! How cathartic would a Term pregnancy and birth be my second time round?! Or would it??? Would I end up feeling guilty for enjoying everything I didn't get to enjoy with my first pregnancy? Would I feel like I was betraying my premmie?? As traumatising as my Neo journey was, I wouldn't want to ever detract from it; because ultimately it is part of who I am now and is deeply woven into my life. I just wish there was a cut and dried answer for all the conflicting questions I have, because I am well aware that my age will soon be against me and my biological clock is ticking – and I may end up regretting the outcome if I don't make a decision soon. The decision to get pregnant the first time didn't take this much consideration – but then again, I didn't know *then* what I know *now*. But despite all my unanswered questions and multitude of concerns, I do have the presence of mind to know that I need to be comfortable in whichever decision we make about expanding our family, because at the end of the day I want it to be for the RIGHT reasons – NOT to just fulfil my unfinished burning desires to experience that sense of pregnant 'fullness' and joyous post birthing baby moon bliss. I need to seriously ask myself, whether I truly DID miss out on so much, and if it IS such a big deal to want to re-enact a 'do-over'… or is what I am feeling just fall-out from all the emotional trauma, both with my premature birth and Post-natal Depression? One thing I DO know for sure - I don't want my son to grow up an only child. But I need to find my centre first.

I saw this simple line on a premmie Facebook site once, and it rings so true – if there is *one* piece of advice I wholeheartedly agree with for new Neo Mum's or for those currently going through it; it is simply this: :

FIND THE JOY IN YOUR JOURNEY.

I love that quote.

If I may offer my humble opinion and advice – look at your Journey this way:

It may not be what you expected or planned or bargained for, but it's yours to own and make of it what you will. Cherish each and every moment and milestone, and don't be afraid or embarrassed to make a big deal out of them. As premmie Mums, it's the little things that mean the most. No-one else will understand the excitement of your baby going down a litre on the Hi-Flo, or the pride you feel when your baby can tolerate an extra Ml of milk per hour.

Take LOTS of photos and hand and footprints. Once a prem hits their stride, they grow and change so much – even every few days. Keep a daily diary. Write your premmie a letter to give to them when their older. Gather information. Keep a treasure box of your premmie's paraphernalia.

Ask a multitude of questions. Get to know your baby's carers – for they will be able to guide you best in getting to really know your precious bundle. And on the days where it all just seems too much and you find yourself beginning to falter – allow yourself to cry and grieve. You don't need anybody's permission to do so.

It's perfectly okay to drop the façade and take some "me" time. You're already a Super Mum – you don't have to prove your worth to anyone. No-one will judge you for it.

And when you do, you will realise how far you and your baby have already come. You ARE more emotionally stronger than you think. And you CAN do this!! And whilst you might not think of it at the time, your birth story is unique and one of a kind and will be worth sharing as something ultra-special in years to come. You and your baby had to fight hard to get where you are today.

Mum's of Neo Premmie twins – you have had to fight TWICE as hard! That's not something to hide. Be proud of it!! Talk about it, share it. All our journeys are so vastly different, but they essentially have one powerful common denominator. I know for myself, that hearing other Neo story's is humbling; and you can identify with certain situations of someone else's experience, even if you yourself didn't go through it quite the same. At the time, you are in pure survival mode and blindly functioning by rote, but once your Neo journey has come to an end, and the adrenaline and hyperactivity has settled down; you can take time to reflect and acknowledge all that you have been through, and give it the validation it deserves.

And perhaps, given time (sometimes MORE time for some, than for others), you will know and appreciate that what you went through was something far greater than those who have 'just a normal Term birth' ; and you may even, one day, understand the magnitude of the sheer beauty and wonderment of what you experienced with your premmie. I say this, because I am now on the healing side of it all, and even though it is still tough, I know it IS possible.

But if you ARE finding it hard to cope post-Neo, REACH OUT. What you have been through was enormous and life changing. Pregnancy, childbirth and new motherhood is no simple feat. And if you are reading this, then it means that you faced it and survived all aspects of it – but if you now find yourself in front of another brick wall that's sapping you of your maternal happiness, it's time to dig a bit deeper to meet these newest adversities head on. Because you CAN do it. You DO have the strength.

Be it in the form of confiding in a trusted family member or friend, your local GP, a registered counsellor or even seeking solace from an online support group – it doesn't matter WHO; just so long as you're not going it alone.

Keeping the lines of communication open is key to staying connected to those around you and rising above what is threatening to bring you down.

Likewise – I urge anyone who feels that they MAY be suffering with Postnatal Depression, to please seek help also. As a fellow Mum who has felt the ravages of PND, I know all too well how overwhelming that suffocating despair feels like.

And how utterly isolated it can make you feel. But this is a time for you to be enjoying your precious baby, and it should be done without being marred by the fears and sadness and desolation that Postnatal Depression harbours.

Find somebody who you are comfortable talking to. Don't let pride get in the way.

Don't be embarrassed. Confront your fears. If you are struggling to cope – don't be afraid to ASK. You do not – and SHOULD not – have to go through it alone.

Sometimes though, the mere offer of help is not enough. For those ladies who are proud women, the extension of support is almost never acted upon. We don't like to ask. We don't like to think we are putting people out. A pro-active approach may be the answer to helping a struggling mum in need. Don't ask – just DO. There might be a bit of an initial protest, but it won't be for too long; and THAT mum will KNOW that your offer of support WAS genuine.

But above all else, remember that suffering from Post-natal Depression is no reflection on you as a mother, or as a person. We are human. And just like technology, the data pack that we are biologically made up of is flawed. But the more that we, as united women, can feel comfortable in helping ourselves and each other and accepting that these things happen for no apparent reason; means that we are empowering ourselves and by doing so, giving ourselves the courage to overcome our fears and adversities.

Giving Postnatal Depression a wider social recognition will hopefully make it better understood by mainstream public – without the reprisals; and the further the reach of acceptance, the stronger the safety net to those women so desperately needing the support.

GLOSSARY OF TERMS USED

NNU - Neonatal Unit

NICU - the ICU component of the NNU

NSCU - the Special Care component of the NNU

ROP - Retinopathy of Prematurity, a condition of the eyes that can cause blindness in babies.

HELLP – stands for H (haemolysis - red blood cell damage); EL (elevated liver enzymes - indicating liver damage); and LP (low platelets in the blood leading to a bleeding tendency). HELLP syndrome can arise at any stage during the second half of pregnancy. Delivery is required for cure of the HELLP syndrome, irrespective of the stage of the pregnancy and maturity of the baby.

PE – Short for Pre-Eclampsia; a pregnancy condition and often a precursor to HELLP Syndrome. Presents itself by high blood pressure, fluid retention and large amounts of protein in the urine.

pPROM - Preterm Premature Rupture of Membranes prior to 37 weeks of gestation. It complicates 2 - 4% of all singleton and 7 - 20% of twin pregnancies and is associated with over 60% of preterm births.

DESAT - short for desaturation, refers to when the infant's oxygen saturation level in the blood drops below the targeted oxygen saturation level.

APNOEA - defined as cessation of breathing by a premature infant that lasts for more than 20 seconds and / or is accompanied by hypoxia or bradycardia. A common occurrence for prem babies due to the brain being immature and it forgets to tell the body to breathe.

BRADY - Short for Bradycardia. When the heart rate is less than 100 beats per minute for more than 10 seconds. Another common occurrence for a prem.

ROP - Retinopathy of Prematurity, a condition of the eyes that can cause blindness in a premature baby.

NEC - Necrotising enterocolitis. A condition where parts of the immature bowel starts to die off due to bacterial infection or as a result of prematurity. The mortality rate of NEC is 20 - 40%. The severity, radiology, management and treatment of NEC are best exemplified by the 'Modified Bell's staging criteria'.

SGA - short for Small for Gestational Age.

CAFHS - stands for Child and Family Health Service

REFERENCES FOR STATISTICAL INFORMATION

Australian Government Institute of Health and Welfare
www.aihw.gov.au

Beyond Blue
www.beyondblue.org.au

The Australian Parenting Website
www.raisingchildren.net.au

Miracle Babies Foundation
www.miraclebabies.org.au

National Premmie Foundation
www.prembaby.org.au

L'il Aussie Prems Foundation
www.lilaussieprems.com.au

Post and Antenatal Depression Association Inc.
www.panda.org.au

Wikipedia
www.wikipedia.org

FACEBOOK SUPPORT GROUPS
That I regularly visit ……….
(most listed below are CLOSED groups, for privacy)

Women Who Have Been There
National Premmie Foundation
Miracle Babies Foundation
L'il Aussie Prems Foundation
Prematurity Awareness
Premature Babies Group Australia
Premmie Support Group
Beyond Blue
Panda SA

If you are struggling and need someone to talk to –

National Perinatal Depression Helpline
1300 726 306

Beyond Blue
1300 224 636

Lifeline
13 11 14